In the Public Interest

Critical Issues in Health and Medicine

Edited by Rima D. Apple, University of Wisconsin–Madison,
and Janet Golden, Rutgers University, Camden

Growing criticism of the U.S. health-care system is coming from consumers, politicians, the media, activists, and health-care professionals. Critical Issues in Health and Medicine is a collection of books that explores these contemporary dilemmas from a variety of perspectives, among them political, legal, historical, sociological, and comparative, and with attention to crucial dimensions such as race, gender, ethnicity, sexuality, and culture.

For a list of titles in the series, see the last page of the book.

In the Public Interest

Medical Licensing and the Disciplinary Process

Ruth Horowitz

Rutgers University Press

New Brunswick, New Jersey, and London

Library of Congress Cataloging-in-Publication Data

Horowitz, Ruth, 1947–
In the public interest : medical licensing and the disciplinary process / Ruth Horowitz.
    p. ; cm. — (Critical issues in health and medicine)
    Includes bibliographical references and index.
    ISBN 978-0-8135-5427-3 (hardcover : alk. paper) — ISBN 978-0-8135-5426-6
(pbk. : alk. paper) — ISBN 978-0-8135-5428-0 (e-book)
    I. Title. II. Series: Critical issues in health and medicine.
    [DNLM: 1. Licensure, Medical—United States. 2. Clinical Competence—United States.
3. Government Regulation—United States. 4. Professional Autonomy—United States.
5. Professional Review Organizations—United States. 6. Public Opinion—United States.
W 40 AA1]
    LC classification not assigned
    362.1068—dc23

                                                                                    2012005097

A British Cataloging-in-Publication record for this book is available from the British Library.

Visit our website: http://rutgerspress.rutgers.edu

Manufactured in the United States of America

Contents

Acknowledgments

Many people provided different kinds of support for this project. My fellow medical board members and their staff from across the country, the staff of the Federation of State Medical Boards, and my colleagues from the Citizen Advocacy Center taught me how to be a public member and what medical boards did. Among the very long list of public members who taught me what a public member could be were Mary Del Long, Susan Spaulding, and Maralyn Turner. David Swankin and Becky LeBuhn of the Citizen Advocacy Center started me on my journey of learning what it takes to become an effective public member. Many members and staff of the Federation of State Medical Boards took me under their wings over the years, especially Lisa Robin, Barbara Schneidman, and Kelly Alfred. There are too many others to mention who helped me out over the years, but I would especially like to thank the members and staff of the boards where I sat who put up with me and all the members and staff from across the country whom I met over the years and with whom I often discussed boards and public participation.

Many board members and staff across the country helped by providing their views on the medical licensing and disciplinary processes, and several colleagues read all or parts of the manuscript and provided very useful comments. Some commented on the entire manuscript at various stages. I would especially like to thank (in alphabetical order) Robert Dingwall, Joel Horowitz, Bunnie and Ed Lehman, Dmitri Shalin, and Mark Yessian. Several of my honors undergraduates provided assistance, including Chloe Anderson, Evan Hasbrook, Laura Pratt, and Danielle Sharon. Lynn Chancer, Kathleen Gerson, Sidney Halpern, Lynne Haney, Josy Ingersoll, and Arlene Skolnik listened to me and provided helpful feedback while I worked through this book's issues, as did Isabelle Baszanger, Henri Peretz, and Maud Simonet, who invited me to try to explain our state-based system of medical regulation to those who are used to national systems of regulation in France and who helped to make my analysis tighter. I would also like to thank Jennifer Dropkin for contributing her excellent copyediting skills. There are many others who contributed greatly to my participation and understanding of medical boards. Thank you.

Abbreviations

AAMC	American Association of Medical Colleges
AARP	American Association of Retired Persons
ABMS	American Board of Medical Specialties
ACCME	Accreditation Council for Continuing Medical Education
ADR	alternative dispute resolution
AG	Attorney General
AHRQ	Agency for Healthcare Research and Quality
AIM	Administrators in Medicine
ALJ	administrative law judge
AMA	American Medical Association
ASPE	Assistant Secretary for Planning and Evaluation, HHS
CAC	Citizen Advocacy Center
CLEAR	Clearinghouse on Licensure, Enforcement, and Regulation
CME	continuing medical education
CMR	comprehensive medical review
COCO	Conference of Consumer Organizations
DO	Doctor of Osteopathy
DOL	U.S. Department of Labor
ECFMG	Educational Commission for Foreign Medical Graduates
Federation Bulletin	former name of the *Journal of Medical Licensure and Discipline*, which later became the *Journal of Medical Regulation*
Federation	Federation of State Medical Boards
FLEX	Federation Licensure Examination
FMA	Florida Medical Association
FSMB	Federation of State Medical Boards
GMC	General Medical Council (UK)
HCFA	Health Care Finance Administration
HCQUIA	Health Care Quality Improvement Act
HEW	U.S. Department of Health, Education, and Welfare
HHS	U.S. Department of Health and Human Services
HMO	health maintenance organization
HSA	Health Systems Agency
IC	investigatory committee
IOM	Institute of Medicine
IPC	impaired physicians committee

IPP	impaired physicians program
JAMA	*Journal of the American Medical Association*
MAG	Medical Association of Georgia
M&M	morbidity and mortality
MD	Doctor of Medicine
MedChi	Maryland Medical Society
NBME	National Board of Medical Examiners
NCHCA	National Commission for Health Certifying Agencies
NCOL	National Council of Occupational Licensing
NCSL	National Council of State Legislators
NPDB	National Practitioner Data Bank
NYPIRG	New York Public Interest Group
OIG	Office of the Inspector General
PRO	peer review organization
PSRO	professional standards review organization
QIO	quality insurance organization
TMA	Texas Medical Association
USMLE	United States Medical Licensing Examination

In the Public Interest

Introduction

Medical Boards and the Public Interest

We know from numerous surveys that most of us are satisfied with our personal doctors. And yet doubts occasionally surface as to whether a doctor did the right thing or put our interests first. How do we know our physicians are competent, ethically fit, and have our best interests at heart? Could a doctor have spotted a tumor before it spread? What do you do if your doctor acts strangely, operates on the wrong body part, reeks of alcohol, or touches you inappropriately?

All such questions involve issues of public interest and trust. Democratic societies develop mechanisms to ensure medical professionals are properly trained and licensed to deliver services to the public. Varying from state to state, those mechanisms have been updated continually in the last forty years in the United States to satisfy new political, economic, and social demands.[1] This book takes a close look at medical licensing and disciplinary boards, institutions designed to decide questions of public interest, and examines the special role that boards play in holding physicians accountable for their actions.

Several other organizations are also charged with the responsibility of monitoring doctors' performance, yet state medical boards are the only organizations authorized to give and revoke permission to practice medicine. Medical societies may deactivate members, but they cannot stop physicians from working. While Peer Review Organizations (PROs, now called Quality Insurance Organizations, or QIOs) conduct overall quality reviews for Medicare and Medicaid programs, they view their mission largely as educational, and, despite a poor review, a doctor can continue to practice. Similarly, liability insurers, who have the right to increase insurance rates for problem doctors, shy away from denying insurance coverage. Health maintenance organizations (HMOs) and hospitals may suspend or remove physicians from their lists, but physicians are free to continue their practice elsewhere.[2] Informal evaluations and reprimands by colleagues are effective during training, but once a physician is credentialed and licensed, the collegial review process is rare and lacks efficacy.[3] Specialty boards generally require updating of credentials at specified intervals, but doctors do not need to be board certified to practice medicine. Aggrieved patients have the option of taking complaints to courts, and successful malpractice suits can bring financial relief, but they do little to protect other patients from incompetent or negligent physicians.[4]

Only licensing and disciplinary boards have the power to restrict doctors' practices, order additional training, or revoke licenses. Things are further complicated by the fact that "malpractice" as defined by the courts differs from the definitions of "medical misconduct" inscribed in medical practice acts that created medical licensing and disciplinary boards at the end of the nineteenth century. A single error may constitute "malpractice" without being considered "medical misconduct," the latter referring to patterns of poor practices or sometimes a single incident rising to the level of "gross misconduct." "Medical misconduct" is a broadly defined category covering acts of negligence, incompetence, sexual impropriety, fraud, felony convictions, and substance abuse and sales, with specific definitions varying from state to state.

The latest push to balance public and private mechanisms for regulating the medical profession is a departure from an early emphasis on professional self-monitoring. The early twentieth-century efforts to mix state and civil procedures created ample opportunities for boards to evade public scrutiny by working behind closed doors with board members selected by professional associations. But boards had the authority of the state to grant and revoke licenses to practice. The scene grew more diversified and transparent starting in the late 1970s when public members were added in most states, open meetings were encouraged, and disciplinary results were made public. Transparency varies considerably among states.[5] Some boards, lodged inside state bureaucracies, have state employees with decision-making authority, while others work independently from the state, relying on staff hired by and answerable directly to the board. Most fall somewhere in between.

Today each state in the nation and Washington, DC, has a board, although fourteen states have separate MD (Doctor of Medicine) and DO (Doctor of Osteopathy) boards, and one has separate licensing and disciplinary boards.[6] While licensure fees fund boards, most are underfunded, in part because state agencies use physician-licensing fees to pay for other budget items. The responsibilities granted to the boards vary—most issue licenses and mete out discipline; some are charged with the responsibility of writing policies and developing regulations. Mostly, boards have between seven and fifteen members working fifteen to twenty-five days a year. The ground shifts often as legislatures tinker with medical practice acts in response to board requests or publicized crises.

National surveys have shown that Americans do not know much about licensing boards.[7] When asked which organization protects them from incompetent physicians, almost half said they did not know, and only 8.7 percent pointed to state medical boards. This is not surprising given that, for much of their history, medical boards operated as a direct extension of the profession and with little input from the general public. More recent data from a *Consumer Reports* survey showed that about 19 percent of their sample said they knew to report hospital errors to their licensing boards. The respondents further said they wanted access to federal data (from the National Practitioner Data Bank) on malpractice, hospital privileging, and licensure actions (88 percent); wanted easy access to state licensure actions with a description of the doctors' problems (79 percent); and wanted to read patients' complaints against doctors, but with the patient's identity omitted (81 percent).[8]

As long as the public did not question physicians' self-regulation, few questions arose.[9] But public trust in professionals eroded, and evidence mounted that physicians' agendas may be at cross-purposes with the public interest.[10] Calls demanding more state and public oversight grew steadily, and by the 1970s, ignoring them was no longer an option.[11] The view of the medical profession prior to 1970 as uniformly committed to the common good changed in light of the realities of a profession increasingly run as a big business and blatant errors making headlines.[12]

Public awareness of physicians' mistakes and errant behavior has grown. Long waits for appointments and treatment, the mounting costs of health care, the closing of hospitals, and stories of doctors' mistakes, predatory sexual behavior, and drug abuse appear regularly in the news. Television no longer portrays doctors as selfless practitioners, as it once did in the 1950s and 1960s. Now they are more likely to appear arrogant and flawed, as anyone who has watched television dramas like *ER*, *House*, or *St. Elsewhere* knows. In 1999, a notorious case, highlighting the profession's failure to self-regulate, became the subject of James Stewart's book *Blind Eye*. A medical school did not discipline Dr. Michael Swango after a felony conviction, and a hospital failed to investigate a string of suspicious deaths. It took time to connect the dots, but eventually Dr. Swango went to jail for murder. When in 1999 the Institute of Medicine released its report on extensive medical errors titled *To Err Is Human*, it became front-page news. Atul Gawande, a surgeon, described learning on patients and errors common among doctors in his widely read series of essays published in the *New Yorker*.[13] Journalists began to spotlight the operation of licensing and disciplinary boards. One notable case in Massachusetts involved a psychiatrist engaged in an unprofessional relationship with her deeply disturbed patient who committed suicide; the doctor surrendered her license, and the inquiry showed that the board failed to act expeditiously. Two books on the incident followed.[14]

This book examines the work of organizations legislated to control who can practice medicine, the balance of public and private interests in regulatory activity, and the manner in which public interests are safeguarded, and sometimes subverted, by those involved in medical board work.[15] The discussion reflects more than fifteen years of my work as a public member on two medical boards, as well as my observations made during the annual meetings of the Federation of State Medical Boards (FSMB, or Federation), the annual meetings of the Citizen Advocacy Center (CAC), an organization that helps to train and educate public members, and my time spent sitting on the CAC board. I also attended public meetings of two additional boards to acquire different vantage points. I have made the standard precautions here to ensure privacy and compliance with regulations governing research with human subjects. Confidentiality is critical to this work. To assure confidentiality I do not use the names of people I observed or spoke with, nor do I make any references that might reveal any state identities.[16] My primary focus is on the ways medical boards frame their discussions and the conditions under which public members can participate effectively in decision-making processes.[17]

It is also important to note that I have waited a long time to write this book, and the specific processes have continually evolved. Not only have state board setups and procedures changed radically over time, but today they also differ considerably by state and continue to change. To understand why medical boards failed to protect the public, how they are doing it better today, and how to strengthen them further, we need to explore their history—to look at how the practice of medicine shifted from market control, to a profession that self-regulated at the end of the nineteenth century, and, when challenged in the 1970s, to a system open to democratic controls, with multiple voices participating with legal mechanisms constraining the privilege to practice medicine.[18]

While disapproving words from colleagues contribute to social control, the movement toward institutionalized forms of control raises new questions.

As Rosemary Stevens put it, "What is and should be the relationship of the profession of medicine and the public interest? Who defines this 'interest'? Is it definable at all? If so, by whom?"[19] We need to understand why particular forms of control develop and change in order to understand the strength and weakness of the different voices now involved in the processes. In the market-based system of the nineteenth century, the mantra was "Let the buyer beware." Early twentieth-century self-regulation allowed the regulated group to determine a common good for others. As it is currently construed, the system approximates a deliberative or participatory democracy that blends voices of medicine, law, and the public in deciding what a common good is. Medical boards today generally employ a hodgepodge of talk in their deliberations, variously highlighting rehabilitation, legal standards, and public protection. In deciding discipline, sometimes they focus on the doctor, at other times on his or her conduct, and less frequently on the patients.[20] Each method of social control raises issues concerning the nature of public good and the proper way of determining its content.

Today, while appeals to public interest and public protection are made during board deliberations, it is far from clear what constitutes common good in any particular case or who is authorized to speak on behalf of the public. A doctor's drinking habits may be excused on grounds that he fell on hard times after a death in the family and should be helped. The question of continuing harm that a drinking physician poses to the public may be sidestepped just as it can be used as rationale for removing the problem physician from practice. A doctor educated in a foreign country could be denied a license to practice in a given jurisdiction with a casual reference to the fact that there are enough physicians working in this area, leaving open the question as to whether board members were motivated by concern for the quality of the physician or by growing competition. Toughening the exam requirements for new physicians may weed out less-qualified doctors, but it may decrease the number of physicians.

When everybody styles themselves as experts on what the public good is, the public interest is likely to be underarticulated, the ramifications of a particular decision is likely to be unexplored, and the reference to common good often then masks vested interests of particular groups. Doctors are trained to make an expert call in cases involving technical medical issues, but they cannot legitimately claim particular expertise to pass judgment on a problem physician's character or to assess the balance of anticipated and unanticipated consequences that a particular board holding will set in motion. It is in this context that the movement to add public members to medical boards started.

First appointed to a medical board in the 1960s in California, public members are now a standard feature of medical boards in all but three states.[21] The idea that the public should have its own representatives on a board is generally accepted today, but it was once controversial, and vestiges of the old debates about the need for their presence can still be heard. By examining the participation of public representatives, we can gain insight into a larger set of issues confronting our technologically driven society, which has grown increasingly dependent on expert judgment, and which has a potential for undermining the ability of communities to govern themselves.

I argue that the problems public members encounter in their board work epitomize the difficulties a deliberative democracy as a whole faces at a time when people cannot readily get to a public square and debate the policies affecting their lives. Our nation's ideals call for informed citizens to deliberate on public issues and elect representatives to governing bodies. These ideals are much harder to uphold in a technologically advanced environment in which public policy has grown so complex that it often defies comprehension by lay persons, and this creates the need to bring in technical experts, a role that developed at the end of the nineteenth century. Experts usually define themselves as public servants, but they can also cater to special interest groups that look for ways to benefit their members, not necessarily the public as a whole.[22]

"Managerialism" is a philosophy that rationalizes the need to take major decisions away from the public, to farm them out to political and scientific elites trained in a particular area. Embedded in a government bureaucracy, managerial decision makers came increasingly to dominate the regulatory landscape beginning in the mid-nineteenth century. The managerialism that governed occupations was distinct from large-scale bureaucracies. Occupational communities have their own bureaucratic dimension, but differ in form from typical government bureaucracies. The managerial revolution continued into the 1960s when a countermovement sought to rein in technocrats and bring communities back into the decision-making process. At that time, the need to combine technical expertise with direct community oversight became evident to many social scientists and grassroots community organizers who came to realize that "managerial science" alone could not ensure the protection of public-interest assessments. The issues that come up in licensing board deliberations illuminate the conflict over the proper place of expert knowledge and grassroots activism, as well as the need to clarify the notion of the common good and increase the range of voices engaged in articulating public interest.[23] These issues arise in the broader society and not just because of changes within the profession; they are examined in this book.

Chapter 1, "Public Member, Researcher, and Public Sociologist: The Genesis of a Project," shows how some boards, differently linked to civil society and state bureaucracies, operate at the turn of the twenty-first century through my experiences as a public member. Drawing on those experiences and as a sociologist, I discuss the history of the present project, the role I assumed as a public sociologist, the problems I faced combining these roles, and questions my experiences raised about the history of boards and about the institutional setups that encourage or subtly discourage public members from peeling off the protective veneer of professional knowledge.

Chapter 2, "How Licensure Became a Medical Institution," examines the transformation from a free market in therapeutics to an occupation regulated by state legislatures that, at the end of the nineteenth century, laid down the framework for determining what the practice of medicine was and who could practice it, along with many other largely health related occupations as big businesses began to dominate the marketplace.[24] Market forces were replaced by "professionalism" as the best way to safeguard the public good, although the public was far from sure about the wisdom of this idea. The rhetoric of public good, I try to show, was harnessed to the cause of licensing and helped physicians secure their credentials as a profession whose members were to act as public servants mindful of a larger public good. The establishment of medical boards played a key role in this process. But during seventy years of medical board activity, the profession insulated itself from public scrutiny, claiming exclusive right and knowledge to define the public good in medical practice.

Chapter 3, "Public Participation: The Federal Bureaucracy Starts a Public Dialogue," shows how seeds of change were planted when the question arose of federal government accountability for Medicare and Medicaid payments to doctors rather than other health-care providers who might do it for less. Federal government efforts were spurred by criticisms from physician board members, public-interest activists, and academic researchers who made the case that the medical profession was far from working toward a public good.[25] The American Medical Association (AMA) declined to mount forceful opposition to federal government agencies when they urged greater board accountability and proposed to add public members. Public participation threatened the autonomy of the medical profession, but the AMA counted on public participation working largely to legitimate board actions in the public eye, while regarding the threat of national licensure as more significant.

Chapter 4, "The State, the Media, and the Shaping of Public Opinion," focuses on state-level debates over the role of public members, the increasing involvement of government actors, and the emboldened media. My thesis is that development of a new constituency for board work among public-interest groups ran parallel to the mounting challenges the profession faced from market forces and new assertiveness on the part of the government. Board members' claims that the licensing process protected the public interest came under attack. In this chapter I also show that, despite national efforts, wide variation remains—for example, in the percentage of public members, the degree of transparency, and the extent to which boards remain in civil society or are incorporated in state bureaucracies. Local medical societies continue as an influence despite the fragmentation of national medical organizations over new issues.

Chapter 5, "Rhetorics of Law, Medicine, and Public Interest Shape Board Work," discusses the parameters of the medical-professional, legal-administrative, and public-civic domains brought to bear on disciplinary cases. Each of these discursive domains has an interest group supporting its cause and trying to channel the discussion accordingly. No board relies exclusively on one particular form of talk, discursive domains do not necessarily conflict, and participants do not always stick to one domain. The civic domain often appears to be the weakest one, for the role of public members has never been clearly articulated, whereas legal and medical discourses are well codified.

Chapter 6, "Medical and Legal Discourses in Investigatory Committees," takes up the first two stages of the disciplinary process. I argue that both medical and public members possess unique and valuable skills; their ways of talking and arguing bring to light different facets of each case, and that special effort must be made to deploy those resources. This chapter illuminates how public participation is affected by the domains of law and medicine. The dominant domain shapes the discourse and provides variable space for public participation. I explore why public members have a hard time finding their own voices. My contention is that legal discourse leaves more room and provides more resources for public members to make their case but does not always work to protect public interest.

Chapter 7, "Hearing and Sanction Deliberations: Transparency and Fact Construction Issues," raises the issue of balance between transparency and privacy, along with the dilemmas posed by each. Although increased transparency provides a better understanding of and increased accountability for board actions and curtails some aspects of the medical-professional discursive domain, it also sensationalizes details of high-profile, difficult cases, and it complicates deliberations on the proper sanctions, especially when the audience behaves uncivilly.

Chapter 8, "Democratic Deliberation and the Public Interest," proposes a corrective to Freidson's theory of professional self-regulation as the best model of social control—that of deliberative democracy. I argue that it was not just consumerism and managerialism that led to failure of self-regulation but the social closure of the profession. While necessary in principle, professional autonomy may insulate practitioners from the needs of the public. I show how we can improve deliberative democracy on medical boards, making the case that while medicine has held much of the discursive power over the disciplinary process, law provides a strong counterweight by making public voices heard. I propose that increased transparency is necessary, that civic groups at the national and local levels are essential in the policy process, and that boards should continue to operate at the intersection of the state with civil society and include strong state, public, and professional actors.

Chapter 1

Public Member, Researcher, and Public Sociologist

The Genesis of a Project

My position as a board member evolved over time. I started as a citizen doing my civic duty, a member of society who happened to be a sociologist, invited to serve first on Board A, then Board B. With the passage of time, my role as a committed intellectual made itself felt, and I slowly became an organic public sociologist in dialogue with public advocacy groups and medical profession-als.[1] As my roles merged, the multiple vantage points fed back and forth, providing me a richer understanding. I was also in a position to cultivate a heightened reflexivity in understanding the social world and my place in it. Each position raised a special set of issues.

Working for an organization educating public members thrust me into the role of organic public sociologist and underscored the need to think more systematically, which in turn also activated my skills as a professional social scientist on Boards C and D. While navigating my various roles and engaging in dialogues with board members, I saw the connection between routine board deliberations and general procedures of deliberative democracies and the need to understand the changes that were occurring. The fact that I had to juggle multiple identities sensitized me to the meaning of committed citizenship in a democratic community and the difficulties we all face while trying to live up to the ideals of democratic participation.

As a Public Member

I faced different realities when I joined first Board A and then, more than ten years later, Board B, each one reflecting different board setups, institutional history, and my own experience. Officially under the aegis of a state bureaucracy, Board A was actually quite independent from the state, except that a deputy attorney general was required to prosecute its disciplinary cases. At the time of my appointment in the late 1980s, the board had only a part-time secretary and offered no formal training for its members. I spent eight years serving on this board, which licensed about two thousand physicians. The state's medical practice act generally followed the Federation of State Medical Boards (FSMB) Model Practice Act of the 1980s, and yet it was far from being an exemplary modern board and sometimes seemed to resemble the boards from the 1950s and 1960s.[2]

Board B worked within a state bureaucracy, and its well-trained staff tried valiantly to improve board performance, educate members, and live up to its mission of protecting the public. It had state-employed staff lawyers and investigators to develop and prosecute cases, but it was difficult to ascertain what happened to reports dismissed by staff and unseen by board members. This state licensed more than fifty thousand physicians.

By the time I was appointed to Board B, I was an experienced public member who had participated in several national committees of the FSMB and had some reputation. The difference between Boards A and B was significant, manifested in their structures, interactions between the participants, and general philosophy. No two boards are quite alike, yet some problems boards face and the solutions they work out are common. Board A can serve as an example of an underfunded, traditional board without strong ties to a state bureaucracy, whose members often catered chiefly to the medical community and did all the work. What they seemed to be doing was peer review. Board B was reasonably well-funded, had a large staff, and was deeply embedded in the state bureaucracy with staff who had some decision-making authority and handled much of the regulatory work. The second board had three foci—the medical community, the state bureaucracy, and the public. This board's work did not seem like peer review; there were too many lawyers present.

Degrees of Being an Outsider

When I first received a call from the governor's appointment secretary asking me to become a public member of Board A, I had little idea what the board did or who the members were. The appointment secretary had no information about board activities or time commitment. I contacted the public member who told me the work was interesting and entailed a monthly board meeting that started at 4 P.M. and often stretched until 11 P.M. Each member conducted investigations of doctors who were singled out by various parties (patients, health-care personnel, or insurance companies) as deficient in some respect and under investigation for violations of the practice act. If the charges were seen as warranted, board members sat on panels of three, advised by a deputy attorney general, to hear the cases. Once the hearing was completed, the entire board discussed the sanction.

I accepted the invitation, even though I was unsure about the time I would need to invest in learning about the board and actively participating and had little understanding of what was going on with the board or what the state's medical practice act was. I did not realize that members did all board work, which included typing letters to complainants, persuading the attorney general to get a subpoena, visiting a doctor's office to get records, interviewing doctors and complainants, and holding hearings that lasted anywhere from one to seventeen days. Many policy issues required additional time and skills, as we had to communicate with other health professions, the medical society, public-interest groups, the media, and the legislature.

When I arrived at my first meeting, ten of the thirteen members were already seated, and the board president asked who I was. I told him I was the new public member, and he handed me an agenda and introduced me to the others, most of whom were significantly older than I. The other women present were a senior physician board member and a part-time secretary who reviewed licensure applications and took notes at meetings. Robert Derbyshire found few women on the boards in the late 1960s.[3] The president suggested I come to his office before the next meeting so he could explain what the board did.

That first meeting began with a waiver hearing of a foreign-trained physician denied a license after failing to obtain the state-defined requisite of seventy-five points on the basic science section of the three-part national FLEX exam.[4] His overall average was well above seventy-five. I knew nothing about FLEX or what score was required. I learned later that foreign medical school graduates had to meet different requirements than U.S.-trained doctors and that passing scores varied among the states. Most states required an overall average of seventy-five, but this state required seventy-five on each section. The physician appeared well qualified to me as he had trained, after practicing for about fifteen years abroad, in several prestigious U.S. university hospitals and was on the faculty of a nationally renowned hospital. He had a job waiting for him in our state in a subspecialty. After he made his plea and several board members asked questions about his qualifications, we went into executive session to discuss the case. I thought his training and a faculty appointment overcame his deficiency of less than one point on one part of an exam, but since I had no idea about the standards at the time, I felt too intimidated to express my opinion.

It appeared that the board was ready to vote against him. The deputy attorney general, who advised the board, reminded us that the law provided an exemption only if the doctor practiced in an "underserved" locality. I felt conflicted and, not knowing what to say, abstained when others voted against his licensure. After the meeting I asked whether doctors out of medical school for many years could pass the basic science section. Several admitted they were rusty. After several such cases we brought our standards in line with the majority of states.

Board members often rejected the "majority of states do it this way" argument, relying instead on the "we do it this way" or "when I was in med school" language of personal experience. The logic made little sense to me and made even less sense when, several meetings later, someone made an argument that a doctor who seemed to be far less educated than the first doctor should be granted a waiver because he was planning to practice in an "underserved" area. Why should some people get less-qualified doctors, I wondered? And what would stop them from moving around the state once they secured a license? The answer to this latter question was that nothing would stop them from moving. If exams measured minimum required competency, why would any state accept lower scores, why did the exemption apply only to "underserved areas," and why were extra training, demonstrated good practice, or outstanding educational credentials not legitimate justifications for an exemption?

Thanks to my talk with the board president, I got a better sense of the board's agenda by our second meeting, but it took time to fathom some of the less obvious rules. Members relied heavily on medical jargon and dropped references to medical diagnoses or treatment options that I could not follow. I was not sure how important it was for me to understand the particular medical diagnosis or terms. It was hard to figure out who made more sense.

The board president gave me my first case to investigate during the second meeting. Many cases under review, I discovered, involved patients' concerns over billing, poor physician communication skills, using or selling drugs, or sexual boundary issues, but the case I received had a clear medical component, which I could not evaluate. The board president suggested that I call the physician to obtain patient records and take them to a specialist. I called and, using my title, "Doctor," asked for the charts of the complainant. He yelled "Never," "Call my lawyer," and hung up the phone. I shuddered as I held the phone, partly from anger, partly from fear. There was nothing in the statutes that protected patients from an offensive physician, not even a private letter of warning. I felt sympathy for the patient's frustration. For a hearing, the doctor's behavior had to rise to the level of gross negligence or incompetence.

I obtained the charts from a second doctor seeing the patient and asked a specialist to help me assess whether the doctor met the standard of care. He claimed the technical care was excellent, and with no way to second-guess him, I had to go along. The case was closed, and I informed the complainant. This first investigation took me more than two full days; the investigation from the time the report was filed until it was resolved took about five months. Neither fellow board members nor I had ever been trained to do our job—constructing cases so they could be heard by a panel.

My third meeting remains vivid in my memory. I could not find my colleagues in the room where we were usually scheduled at 4 P.M. Half an hour later, when nobody showed up, I ran around the capital looking in the state office buildings where I thought the board might be. Something pushed me to check the restaurant where we adjourned after brief public sessions following our first meetings. Perhaps no public sessions or licensure hearings were scheduled, and everyone went directly to the restaurant. As it turned out, the board members had ordered their dinners and drinks in that restaurant. No one had bothered to explain that if no public sessions were held, the entire meeting would be conducted at a restaurant. While we discussed the cases before us, we sat balancing a five-inch-thick packet on our laps containing the meeting agenda, the reports of misconduct, and the summary of licensing actions. It was difficult to read some of the complainant reports, for many were hand-written, and the copy machine was of poor quality. Every month the board president assigned board members new cases to investigate, and all reported on the progress made on open cases. Each doctor applying for licensure was interviewed by two physician board members, which was then discussed and voted on by the entire board. We each paid for our dinners and drinks. I later learned that we were paid fifty dollars for each of ten meetings a year, but that I would be spending fifteen to twenty-five days per year conducting board-related business. We saw everything that came to the board, yet it was apparent that no one could keep track of it all.

When I left that first board, it still did not have a toll-free telephone number to receive complaints, a computer system, an Internet site, or a full-time lawyer assigned to assist the review process. I thought I was done with licensing boards once I moved, but when the call came to join a new board, I changed my mind. It was by comparing Board B with Board A that I realized how lacking in resources Board A was and how much difference the presence of lawyers, outside experts, and professional investigators could make. Board B had excellent support staff and administrative systems—trained investigators (medical and others), staff medical experts, probation supervisors, computerized systems of complaint tracking, staff attorneys (prosecutors), and administrative law judges (ALJs). Located within a reasonably well funded state agency, a nonphysician administrator with substantial statutory authority dealt with supervising impaired physicians, investigations, case construction, probation, and the board unit. The board unit had a president, an advisory group (appointed by the president), and investigatory and hearing committees made up of three, one of whom had to be a public member.

My introduction to the second board was in sharp contrast to my earlier experience. At the annual meeting of the FSMB, I met several board members who told me they wanted experienced public members. The staff worried when they discovered that I had registered as a member of a different political party than the governor, but that was no different from the situation in the other state. Some governors tend to favor public representatives from their own party, and several public members I met at national meetings were not reappointed when a new governor with a different political affiliation was elected. Board staff invited nominated members to their annual two-day training marathon. We received a well-organized packet explaining how the board operated and what we were expected to do at the meeting. When my appointment came through several months later, I was put on a disciplinary hearing panel immediately. Before the hearing, staff provided packets with the charges. I received specific instructions on how to find the meeting and found a sign with my name on the table and a comfortable chair, unlike the metal folding chair I grew accustomed to on Board A.

Looking back, I realized that Board A was still transitioning to a framework that would be dominated by disciplinary review. Its structure resembled that of many other boards in the late 1980s when boards struggled to understand how to manage disciplinary cases and obtain and use legal tools. Board A used legal procedures for disciplinary hearings, but cases rarely made it that far. Board members had to do everything themselves, despite lack of training and varied enthusiasm. Board B had staff members who did all the leg work and had the final say on some of what was done. The entire disciplinary process was framed by law.

Investigations: Medical Language and Voice

Most cases under review are dismissed, or an informal disciplinary outcome is reached, or a settlement is achieved in the course of investigations and investigatory meetings, which is why the investigative phase of the process is so important. When I first joined Board A, it was reasonably easy to see the cases about which I could form an independent opinion and others where I could only say, "I feel something is going on." In cases of sexual abuse, alcohol or drug dependency, or illegal sales, I felt confident I could analyze the information and frame an argument that might resonate with other members. When it came to medical quality-of-care cases, I had a hard time framing sensible questions. At the investigatory stage, we generally relied on the expertise of board members. If the case involved a specialty far outside the specialties of board members, the physicians on the board would ask a friend or colleague to volunteer as an expert. That was how my first case was handled. Reliance on a member's impressions made it difficult for a public member to ask informed questions when the board members would say something like, "Well, those things happen."

In my experience on Board A, informal interactions sometimes created a space for potential influence, but it was difficult to affect the trajectory of disciplinary cases. During investigatory discussions, I was asked if I understood an issue or found explanations satisfactory. This might have been my colleagues' way of handling situations with which they were not completely comfortable, or it might have been a way to co-opt me, but such solicitations gave me an opening to express my views, especially when I found explanations less than persuasive. I noted that investigations sometimes took a new turn when I raised questions and expressed unease about decisions to drop cases without further investigation. After my querying, the assigned investigator went back to do more work. I felt that my concerns were taken seriously, even though in the end the complaint was usually judged lacking in merit. My limited knowledge was insufficient to counter a doctor's assessment of cases of questionable medical skills. My markedly different experience on Board B helped me understand what was going on; some organizational and discursive practices encouraged public members' participation.

Before my first investigatory committee meeting on Board B, I spent about eight hours reading the thick files of the twenty-five physicians whose cases were coming up for discussion. Each case included medical charts, interview summaries, expert evaluations, and a summary by staff. We had to decide which should go to hearings, receive a private administrative warning, or be dismissed. When the committee voted a case to a hearing, it recommended parameters to the head administrator so that staff lawyers could negotiate a settlement to avoid a hearing. A few of the cases were the staff's petitions for a "CMR." I had to ask what that meant and was told "comprehensive medical review." In cases that concerned a doctor's office practice and the board had a simple case of negligence and some evidence of more systematic problems, the investigatory committee decided if it had sufficient evidence to ask for a sample of the physician's cases. In a hospital, printouts could be made of all of a physician's cases that list outcomes and complications.

As a nonmedically trained member, I found reading the cases difficult; they were complex and often required medical knowledge. I did not count the number of acronyms I came across in various documents, but my guess is that each packet contained at least thirty abbreviations and medical terms. When I arrived a few minutes before the meeting, I asked if the board would provide me with a medical dictionary. Public members had served on investigatory committees for more than ten years, but no one had asked for one before. Without a basic understanding acquired prior to a meeting, it would be difficult for a public member to raise questions as everyone jumps into the discussion and assumes that others understand technical terms. Some bought medical dictionaries on their own. I jotted down questions to ask or discuss on the front page of each case packet, which I noticed physicians did as well. I was no more medically sophisticated than before, yet with enough information provided beforehand, I felt I could ask specific, sensible questions, with people listening to my queries and comments on negligence and incompetence cases and not just to questions dealing with fraud, drugs, or sexual misconduct.

Senior staff attending investigatory meetings were well prepared to argue the cases and often disagreed among themselves over both medical and legal points. Many arguments about the gravity of the offense considered were heated, with members discussing whether sufficient evidence was available to put it before a hearing panel. Discussions about what the defense would say in a case and whether a panel would accept the evidence were inevitable. At other times the discussion revolved around the medical facts of the cases or a disagreement over the desirable outcome. Several staff had law degrees, and others had medical or nursing degrees. The medical staff and investigators clarified points.

Despite lack of medical training, public members could aid discussion, provided they had enough description of the diagnosis or treatment. Thus I pushed for an administrative warning in a case that did not rise to the level of medical misconduct in the eyes of the other panel members and most of the staff. I was uneasy about the expert who said the doctor's actions remained above the level of minimally acceptable practice on the cases he evaluated, even though the physician under review was cited repeatedly in the past for sloppy work and had to leave one specialty after a number of malpractice cases went against him. The lawyers told the panel that, since this was a new case, we could not overturn an expert's claim that the questionable performance did not rise to the level of misconduct. I left the meeting with a heavy heart, thinking that the doctor was a danger to the public and that we should have given him a private administrative warning. But I could begin to see the importance of legal argument.

Hearings: Similarity of Legal Practices, Variation in Topics

In my eight years on Board A, we very rarely had cases where negligence or incompetence was the central issue. We had diet doctor cases, sexual misconduct cases, and impairment cases, but diagnoses and treatments were never the central issue. On Board B many of my cases involved negligence or incompetence. My first case on Board A took four days spread over about three months—it was hard to reconcile ten people's schedules. Testimony was wrenching; several of the patients cried profusely. Hearings took place in various venues, most of which were not set up as hearing rooms. We sat on folding chairs, often with only a small narrow table separating the panel from the defense team. The prosecutor, who was in the same office as the deputy attorney general advising the panel, sat to one side; the witnesses, straining to face the panel, sat next to the prosecutor. The panel deliberations that followed the hearing gave me confidence I could make independent assessments, as this case required little knowledge of medicine. I organized the evidence before the panel met to make the decision, persuading both doctors to follow my lead. We had no money for transcripts, so the construction of facts was based on our notes. The panel voted that the doctor committed misconduct, recommending revocation of his license.

On Board A the findings of fact by the panel bind the board, but the full board can vote to change the conclusions of law and the panel's recommendation. Although the board did not contest the recommendations in this case, it discussed the facts for an extended period while the hearing panel waited in the hall. I worried that those most sympathetic to the perspective of protecting the public were on the panel and the board would not be sufficiently tough; they voted to revoke.

The typical Board B member sat on one to three cases (normally one to eight days per case) each year. Although an administrative law judge made the legal decisions, rather than the board with the advice of a deputy attorney general, the hearing was similar. But Board B had transcripts, made very detailed findings of fact and conclusions of law, and decided the sanction. I found I had plenty of information with which to form an opinion, even on highly technical medical cases. Not only was I in a position to question witnesses and query the doctors on the panel, I could also ask the panel members to justify the decision to say one expert was more persuasive than the other. I began to see the importance of legal discourses and practices for public participation. These variations became the focus of my analysis.

State Commitment to Public Protection

The lack of resources of Board A suggested a weak state interest in public protection and democracy, as adequate funding and transparency is necessary. Doctors were happy with the low licensure fees, and state government still kept some of the fees, a national complaint.[5] With limited staff and no money for expert witnesses, trained investigators, transcripts, or travel to national meetings, the board remained parochial. It was difficult to ascertain whether this was the result of a legislature that subscribed to a "small government" philosophy, a by-product of the medical society's interest in having an inactive board, or the board's relative invisibility. However, this clearly underscores the importance of the relationship the board had with the state and medical society. How resources affected the public voice became another focus of my research.

Board B had decent offices and hearing rooms, but it had its share of financial and space problems. There was no place for the hearing panel and defense counsel to talk separately, and some of the hearing rooms had glass doors, so anyone could peek through. But at least the chairs were comfortable and the rooms large enough. Most important, Board B had funds to pay for outside experts and investigators with special skills; it takes different skills to investigate sexual misconduct and negligence/incompetence cases. The availability of and performance by outside experts became one aspect of my research. But with a shrinking state budget, training for board members ended.

Lack of state government interest can affect board transparency. About a year after I joined Board A, the local newspaper pointed out that under the sunshine law, public boards should not do business in a private venue. But the state bureaucracy did not make sunshine work. While we moved our meetings from the restaurant to a state building, the room on the second floor was barely large enough for a table to seat the board, the secretary, and the deputy attorney general. Whenever the public and the media attended, the room was overcrowded and sometimes overheated. Dinner arrangements became problematic. If we went out, our deputy attorney general advised, others might suspect we were discussing board business. We ordered pizza. Someone had to lean out the window to wait for the delivery because a state rule dictated the door downstairs had to be locked at five-thirty (no doorbell). We scrounged for cash for pizza and turned out pockets for change for the soda machine.

Meeting in a public place was intended to open the proceedings to the public, but the facilities were inadequate for the purpose, generating frustration and solidarity among board members. Meanwhile, the locked door made it difficult for the public to attend the "open" meeting. On one occasion, before the general use of cell phones, a physician member, late for the meeting, was unable to enter using conventional means (knocking loudly and yelling). Suddenly, a shower of pebbles hit the second-floor window. Below, the board member waited. Should members of the public wish to attend and arrived after five-thirty, they might not want to throw stones at windows. How to make board meetings more open to the public was an obvious question, yet no one was asking. It was up to the media and public-interest groups to raise the issue, which they did; eventually a new location was found.

The failure to send Board A members to national meetings undermined prospects for reform and deprived members of a chance to learn. National meetings were helpful to me to shape my identity as an active public member. After two years on Board A, I attended the second annual meeting of Citizen Advocacy Center's (CAC) educational training conference, where I discovered that my state had fewer resources and staff than others and that many states had private sanctions in place to warn physicians. As a sociologist, I recognized that private sanctions are a double-edged sword with regard to public protection: a private sanction is less costly and is viewed by some as rehabilitative, and the board can put a doctor on notice, but this action may thereby avoid a more serious and warranted action that would better protect the public. In discussion with other public members at meetings, they began to see the dilemmas of private reprimands. That was encouraging, for I saw that an active stance could promote change.

Encouraged by public members at the CAC meeting, I asked to attend a Federation (FSMB) meeting. I paid for the plane ticket and stayed with relatives but persuaded the state to pay for registration. As a voting delegate, I had a special ribbon on my name tag, and each candidate running for office came up to me and tried to convince me to vote for him or her (mostly "him," for only one candidate was a woman that year). Candidates gave me their handouts and a symbolic gift—a tiny bottle of hot sauce or maple syrup, a packet of wild rice, or a small emblem of the state symbol that could be fastened to the badge. States with candidates brought many board members. One board, funded directly by licensing fees, gave a cocktail party with an open bar and elaborate hors d'oeuvres. The event was attended by the entire board and their wives (there were no women on that board), who greeted each person entering the room. Tales circulated of many parties in the past.

Meetings were well attended for two and a half days.[6] Delegates from each board vote on acceptance of committee reports, issues, and officers, then attend a black-tie dinner with the Bierring Lecture, which was given by the president of the American Medical Association (AMA) when I first attended. I was invited to several private parties, and I felt like one of the team. Attending this meeting alerted me to the connections among medical organizations.

Multiple Vantage Points for Understanding

Multiple vantage points are useful for thinking about boards. As I show in this book, media stories about board problems spurred reforms, but seeing them from a member's perspective, I construed the press attacks differently. The media provided the public with information about boards, thus increasing transparency and the potential for a more active public. Nevertheless, as a board member under attack, I felt uneasy in the spotlight. In some cases, especially vociferous and one-sided coverage created solidarity among members, pushing me to over identify with the doctors. Even when Board A was ranked quite highly by *Public Citizen*, a Ralph Nader public-interest group, the headline in the local paper was negative, compelling the legislature to increase public membership to one-third, which prompted some board members to observe that this was more than in other states.

I was surprised by how much relationships with members on Board A mattered to me when a reporter questioned me about board actions after I attended only three meetings; I certainly had no informed thoughts about the process. She asked my views on how the board protected the public from physicians with AIDS. I had not formed a position on the subject, nor had the board spoken of the issue. The reporter then asked what I thought about the handling of a sexual misconduct case that was in civil court, which was dismissed by the board before my appointment. I did not have a sufficient understanding to answer the questions intelligently, and, had I criticized the board's actions publicly, I would have had a hard time building rapport. I kept answering the reporter with "I don't know."

The reporter did not write about our conversation, but during the following weeks, the newspaper began a series on the sexual misconduct case that the board had dismissed and that, according to the press, it mishandled. This attack led me to identify strongly with the board members and take the critique personally, though it was dismissed before I was appointed. I had to find the right balance between building rapport with the board and being able to maintain independent judgment as a public member. Looking back at the press coverage, I can see that sometimes reporters got it right; other times I wondered if the journalist and I had attended the same meeting. As an analyst, I strive to present multiple sides.

Trust and Deliberative Democracy

As a member, a public sociologist, and researcher, I saw the fine line between trust and co-optation. Board members need to have confidence in each other, but too much trust can undermine willingness to question. Deliberative democracy is known to stumble when people take for granted that their leaders will always do "what is right." Rigorous questions, persuasive arguments, and careful monitoring strengthen democratic institutions. Medical board deliberations are an example of deliberative democracy in action, and as such, they thrive on the ability to voice criticism and monitor outcomes, and they wilt when board members—especially appointed to defend the public good—think that doctors always know best. The profession has a powerful voice in defining what patients want and need, and they influence public members' perspectives.[7] Doctors use their expertise to define what the practice of medicine is, what makes a good physician, and what constitutes the safe practice of medicine. Often what they say goes unchallenged. Some trends counteract this excessive trust. Although Americans trust their personal physicians, they are apt to question physician leaders and organizations today.[8] It also matters that patients and patient rights groups have learned some of the language of medicine and have begun to challenge doctors and medicine's definition of illness and treatments.[9]

Some cases and issues require medical knowledge, and committee work necessitates relying on others' judgments. Respect as a basis for trust helps to ensure that deliberations can work among people with unequal resources. By *respect*, I mean evaluation of the willingness of others to listen, explain clearly, make sensible arguments, stay open to others' arguments, and explore issues from a variety of perspectives. In the discussion that follows, I use my experience as a board member, a public sociologist, and a researcher to unravel the relationship between social skills, respect, and trust. My argument is that, while trust in others is essential to board work, it must grow from respect and not derive from social skills or status.

Boards depend on committees to do much of the work, and some members are more knowledgeable in specific areas. Boards should not need to rehash an entire case when asked to decide the sanction because those who heard it have provided sufficient evidence for their findings and have a history of backing their decisions with sensible rationales. Too little trust may lead to overzealous questioning of every decision made by others. It is not uncommon after a committee has made the findings of fact by which the board is bound by statute that other members want to rehear the case and decide the facts for themselves. When a full board changed a panel's recommended disciplinary action, the panel complained. Boards are sometimes reluctant to reaffirm disciplinary actions taken by other states on locally licensed physicians without rehearing a case. I heard members from many states explain that they needed to rehear cases because they did not trust others' opinions. In states where judges heard cases and boards were not bound by judges' findings of fact, board members and administrators told me that boards often changed the findings of fact as members did not trust lawyers. Sometimes physician members did not trust a particular doctor's expertise because they did not know him personally. Conversely, they were at times eager to place their trust in doctors they knew.

Earning respect is difficult and figuring out who to respect is problematic. When I sent back cases for more investigation on Board A, I believed I had a valid point, but nothing changed the outcome. I knew no one and had little idea whose judgment I could trust. I wanted some knowledge of others. When I was driving home close to midnight, two pick-up trucks with gun racks (and guns) surrounded my car and tried to force me off the road. The next month, when one of the physicians asked me to join the carpool, I accepted. Getting to know several members allowed me to feel like I belonged, but I realized I was more likely to accept my carpool buddies' opinion than before. It took me a long time and several national training meetings to see it was their social skills influencing me.

Attendance at the annual FSMB meetings co-opted me at first with all the party invitations. But public members, including myself, tested the Federation waters by asking for a public member's session. We got our wish but were given a room during the lunch hour on Saturday—when everyone either takes off for the afternoon or is enmeshed in politicking for votes. The session was hard to find on the program and the room difficult to locate. The lawyers and executive directors set up programs, but the public members had few resources, and only a handful of public members attended for more than two consecutive years. I began to wonder if I was invited to parties in part because few women attended at that point.

I continued to attend Federation and CAC meetings and often heard, "We trust our doctors." I began to notice how social skills facilitated the development of trust. It was rather common for me to hear from some public members who socialized with physicians that doctors knew what was best for patients. A public member informed me at a Federation meeting of public members that "we like our doctors." She said this to support another public member who complained that the CAC meeting was antidoctor. Another public member added, "Our members are ethical and we never disagree. All board members think alike." A third added, "There is no tension between public members and doctors—they help us out." These public members tend to rely heavily on physicians in decision making. Trust may blind an individual to the need to ask for and make clear arguments necessary for reasoned assessments of cases and issues. It is possible that some public members are easily swayed by "expert" opinions that they are meant to be guarding against. My experience taught me that the confidence these public members expressed in the physicians had something to do with the physicians' social skills. One told me how pleasantly surprised she was when a doctor invited her to travel with him so he could tell her more about the board. Feeling included and being treated courteously are important, but the danger is to mistake social skills for a commitment to protecting the public interest.[10]

At Federation meetings I dined with boards that brought several members. The conversation was lively, and the board members knew each others' interests outside board activities. It was only after I began to pay systematic attention to board social interactions that I concluded that the ability to schmooze could be conflated with the ability to take a critical stance on problem, a problem I was having. Some boards spend several days together, as many as six times a year, and stay together in a hotel. Sometimes spouses accompanied them and spent the day together, joining the group for dinner. During meals, discussions rapidly evolved into discussions of family, travel, movies, or current events, just like a dinner party among friends. Such gatherings provided the opportunities for trust to develop, but such trust was not always conducive to democratic deliberations and mutual criticism.

I faced a moment of truth on Board A when I realized it was virtually impossible for me to persuade my colleagues to hear incompetency and negligence cases, unlike sex or drug cases, and I was developing too chummy relations with physicians, not unlike the ones I observed at meetings where I heard people take for granted the infallibility of doctors' judgments. But, after a very long argument with a medical member, whom I respected, over pending legislation, I felt confident enough about the issue to alert a state legislator. We had several meetings with the legislative subcommittee and compromised, but on cases that involved technical issues where I had to rely on someone else's judgment, I simply did not have the knowledge to ask the right questions that might change the evaluations of the cases. The doctors were probably humoring me by waiting to dismiss the cases where I requested more investigation.

I am not sure when exactly I became a "public" sociologist rather than just a "citizen," but at that moment, I consciously set out to improve my board. I started questioning public members at national meetings when I heard them say "we like our doctors."[11] Few people showed any interest in the fact that I was a sociologist. I was a public member who had been around longer than some, took pains to learn about board work across the country, and tried to be reflexive about the complexities of the role public members play on medical boards. I had the sociological tools to do that, and I began to use them. If I was a public sociologist when I was pushing some public members to think twice about their trust in physicians, then I was also using my public sociology role to analyze the dangers of putting unreserved trust in physicians' expertise and selflessness.

I asked public members attending the Federation public members' meeting what they thought about my writing a book on boards, and I was relieved to learn that they approved of my agenda and offered help. For several years the Federation provided me with address labels so I could send letters to public members encouraging them to attend Federation meetings and the public members' session. After several years of few resources, the Federation began to provide lunch and programming.

To be sure, many public members are not victims of "blind trust." Some talk about developing respect for certain members rather than blanket trust. "It is never 'us against them' in a vote," a public member told me. "Some relations are stronger than others, and I listen to some more than others. I have one doctor to whom I turn for advice whom I really respect." She distinguished among the medical members but learned to see things from the physicians' perspectives too: "They make mistakes and are not gods. They don't have all the answers. People [the public] also have a great sense of entitlement. Public members need to enter into the language of doctors, and that takes education and training. I take it seriously."

Unlike trust based on social skills, respect is derived more from public displays of reasoning skills and sensibilities at meetings, including informal gatherings. Respect has to be earned—both by physicians and public members. As boards are ongoing organizations, members develop reputations. Within a span of several meetings, people can see which members explore several sides of an issue, offer detailed explanations, and are reliable. Members take a measured look at each other and evaluate each others' stances, manners of carrying out a discussion, voting patterns, and so on. When doubts persist as to the merit of the case, members decide whom to tap for advice and information, and this is where trust and judgment play a major, sometimes decisive, part. Both public members and doctors use their impressions of others in determining

who should be questioned carefully and to whom one should particularly
listen. In discussing how she works on a board, one public member explained
to me how she thinks carefully before challenging someone's opinion: "I will
look at a specific member of the board and will say to them 'maybe I've missed
something'—I don't need to be harsh. So that's another thing I use to determine
the fine gray area, but I'll point to someone personally because you know the
members." A new member of a different board explained her situation: "I'm a
virgin at this. At one meeting I felt that this physician should be disciplined
very harshly in this case and none of the doctors agreed with me, but the other
public member . . . is a very successful businesswoman and they really respect
her. She took the lead and she got what she wanted because they really respect
her—that's the dynamics." Another added that reasonable arguments are
necessary to get the respect of others, "not to make any wild statements . . .
then people pay attention."

According to several public members they gain the respect of doctors by
making sensible arguments. One explained to the group: "I received a compli-
ment about how I talked about a case in the full board. One time we were
discussing a case at the board meeting, and one doctor asked who was on it. I
said I was and he replied—'Oh, then it's ok.'" Failure to speak up and take a
stance can prevent respect. Physicians do not value public members who
remain silent as they do not advance board work. Most encourage questions,
but on some boards, members learn to be careful about expressing views
contradicting others.

Administrators' observations provide another perspective on trust and
respect, and several administrators jotted down opinions of public member
participation when I asked them when public members were first appointed in
each state and how many times the legislation had changed. Some expressed
pessimism about the independence of public members because of limited
training, support, and encouragement. Others were more optimistic and saw
neither interest-group voting nor public members as dominated by physicians.[12]
One wrote, "Our public members represent a broad range of professional and
personal backgrounds. They consistently vote their own viewpoints or those of
their constituencies, if any. In eighteen years of 'Board watching' I've never
seen any sign of P.M. [public members] v. M.D. bloc-voting. If P.M.s take the
same side on an issue it is because that is what they believe." This administrator saw the board members as coming to their decisions through independent assessments. A second thought that some public members were even more
independent than others and wrote that public members did not vote as a
block because of "different backgrounds and training, level of preparation for

meetings, bring[ing] in different perspectives, level of understanding on issues." A third explained, "They [public members] are of very different minds. Two of the three have had training through the Consumer [Citizen] Advocacy Center in Washington, D.C. They are both strong voices on the board for consumers, though they sometimes disagree on particular issues. The third consumer member always casts her vote in accordance with the vote of physicians on the board that she respects." Public members are never the majority; they need respect based on their reasonable questions and persuasive skills.

Doctors also make assessments of each other; one said he imitated the types of questions asked by a physician he admired. After a doctor on one board declared that no licenses should be revoked, he was ostracized and, after failing to attend several meetings, was asked to resign. Failure to make sensible arguments and ask reasonable questions may lead to the ineffectiveness of any member.

Staff members, too, need to respect each other to establish trust. One state agency head decided not to issue an emergency license suspension when advised to do so by a board lawyer. The case concerned a doctor's failure to notify a patient of a serious illness. Dizzy, the patient went to the emergency room, where doctors found the patient had been given a toxic dose of medication. The lawyer felt that the agency head would respect her advice the next time she made a recommendation. Respect is necessary, as persuasion is the tool for influencing others' views.

My experiences taught me that the need to develop trust to depend on others' judgments was related in part to the resources available to board members. In the case of Board B, members had few opportunities to develop relationships based on social relations or respect for fellow board members. Although it did not make it easy for public members to feel a part of the board, I felt less need to rely on trust.[13] I listened carefully to arguments during investigatory committee meetings and hearings and developed respect for the opinions of some physician board members, but I did not have to depend heavily on them, as I did on Board A, even for the technical cases. We had experts who were not board members and contested hearings with two sides articulated and case details presented. I could listen to arguments and ask questions. I did not have to confront a board member's judgment as on Board A without enough information to ask a reasonable question. I used this insight both in talking with other public members and in developing my analysis of the different board discourses. I wasn't a doctor and could not make an independent assessment on incompetence or negligence cases without an expert. "Something smells fishy" is not a strong enough argument to carry the day.

Independent experts were critical to the process, but Board A did not use them often. Board B did, and I was able to ask much more informed questions. What created the differences among boards? Members were not that different.

As a Researcher

I also interacted with two additional boards that I anticipated to be different from Boards A and B. I hypothesized that the degree of independence from a state bureaucracy mattered for public-member participation, but I was unsure why, except that I thought that independent boards were likely to be closer to the medical societies. Board C was an independent board; it collected its own fees, hired its own staff, and operated outside a state bureaucracy. Board D was located in a small underfunded state, and while linked to a state bureaucracy, it worked more independently than Board B and less independently than Board A. Board D was responsible for about the same number of physicians as Board A and worked hard to be innovative. Invited to attend Boards C and D, I had a chance to talk casually to their members between public meetings. Both were "hands-on" boards with members involved in almost all aspects of the process. Board members saw most of the reports that came in and followed them through the disciplinary process.

Board C hired its own staff and had better resources than many others—advanced computer systems and a senior staff member sat with new board members during first meetings to explain what was going on. They met for several days in a row, and committees met during months when the board did not. The investigatory committees heard the presentation of many cases, and a constant parade of doctors arrived for interviews. The full board sat for several hearings, directed by the board president, during a single day in a public session and decided the outcomes the next day. Coffee and cookies were always available, and lunch was served. In the evening board members dined together, often with spouses. The board covered the members' dinners, travel, honoraria, and hotel.

The small state staff of Board D played multiple roles and had tiny offices with state-issued furniture and worn carpets. Senior staff spent a good deal of time delivering papers. The board met once a month. Investigatory and licensing committees met at least one other day per month. The investigatory panel decided which cases involved unprofessional conduct, if proven in a formal hearing. Medical staff presented cases, outside experts were seldom involved, and a committee often interviewed the accused physician. When the investigatory panel found misconduct and no settlement was achieved, a panel of three board members heard the case over several days to assess the evidence and make a finding of unprofessional conduct. The entire board decided the sanction. Board D members received no compensation; staff made coffee for the long meetings, and training was limited. I followed each of these boards for about a year.

As a researcher, I was trained to stand back; as a public sociologist and public member, I learned to take a stance and weigh in. It was difficult not to form opinions on cases when I was in the audience. As a participant I often jotted notes to keep track of the discussion for purposes of persuasion and decision making. I could only summarize at the end of the day. As an observer of public meetings I was able to concentrate on note taking as well as observing subtler communication patterns. Sometimes it was hard to keep up with the fast flow of board interactions.

As a Researcher, Board Member, and Public Sociologist

While I can now categorize my position as public member, public sociologist, or researcher, my role was constantly changing depending upon the place, the people, and what was going on while observing and participating in board work. Keeping apart my identities as public member, expert, public sociologist, and researcher was difficult. The identity that was most salient depended on the situation, and sometimes I had to negotiate the identity in question. It is not like one can entirely turn off one's sociological perspective while acting as a board member. Whatever identity I envisioned for myself, others were likely to see me differently at times. By the time I began as a researcher, I had a reputation as a board expert. Interestingly, I was often asked for my opinion as someone with extensive experience serving on and working with various boards. What physicians seemed to want was a "public sociologist." I certainly could not play the naive observer, as I had in research projects in the past; everyone had questions to ask me, and as a public sociologist, I felt free to share my thoughts on policy issues and organizational matters. We talked about the pros and cons of national licensure requirements, of the structures of review processes, of problems and opportunities public participation creates for boards, and of the limits of transparency. But then the ability to play multiple roles and place oneself in the shoes of others is critical to a deliberative democracy.

My experiences as a board member, public sociologist, and researcher led me to ask a variety of questions. Both as a board member and as a researcher, I needed to understand what was going on, but for different reasons. As a member, I wanted to be the best public member I could be, which first and foremost meant understanding the board. This led me to ask about what my role should be. When was the right time to take a stand against the entrenched majority opinion, engage the legislature, or talk to the media? How could I, as a public member, untrained in medicine, take an independent position on complex medical issues? What should I do to help a board reach an informed decision on where the public interest lies? As a sociologist, I needed to stand back and look at the way decisions were made on different boards and whose voices were heard at the table.

My intuition when I switched boards was that I could participate more fully on Board B than on Board A. But until I stepped back as a researcher and sociologist, I did not realize how different the talk was in the deliberative process depending upon the board. Professional groups coalesce around their members' need to control their work environment, maximize income opportunities, and secure their members' status in society. To achieve these objectives, professionals develop a form of talk or professional discourse highlighting their members' specialized knowledge that only highly trained practitioners possess. The more successful professionals are in developing their own language, the more they are able to maintain self-regulation and determine the public interest for others. Barriers to public members' effective participation have been high, a formidable one being the medical talk that dominates board deliberations and often intimidates nonprofessionals. The medical/professional discourse is not the only one structuring board discussion. With disciplinary cases emerging at the center of board work, the legal-administrative discourse gained a foothold in some board deliberations, often providing an important counterbalance to the once-dominant medical reasoning on disciplinary cases, as was the case on Board B.

The civic/public discourse is one more form of talk increasingly heard on medical boards that helped refocus the discussion on the patient and public protection. Compared to medical and legal reasoning, public discourse is less organized. Its natural constituency—the general public—is hard to mobilize, its interests are underarticulated, and its representatives are often hampered by lack of training. I began to ask how the three forms of discourse developed and how they affected board disciplinary processes.

I realized that I needed to focus on the interplay among three groups of players shaping board deliberations, each one championing a particular kind of discourse—medical, legal, or public. My discussion is based on the premise that modern board work is a form of democratic deliberation that produces a legitimate outcome, acceptable to the community, when all parties involved manage to transcend their immediate interests, take the role of the other, and effectively articulate their points of view.

John Dewey, George Herbert Mead, and Jürgen Habermas are among the modern thinkers who have highlighted the centrality of public discourse to democratic society. According to their views, democratic deliberation achieves its end when (1) all participants have a voice,[14] (2) everyone says what he or she believes, (3) no relevant issue is left out,[15] (4) participants use persuasion rather than authority to win an argument, (5) every issue is examined from multiple perspectives,[16] and (6) deliberation remains civil even when it is emotionally charged.[17] The deliberative process presupposes the freedom to ask questions and the right to receive relevant information. Those partaking in this process must try to persuade as well as remain open to being persuaded.[18] The theory of deliberative democracy predicates its success on the equality of all participants, yet in practice, the participants rarely come to the table with equal resources allowing them to make a forceful argument.[19]

I invite readers to join me in exploring how occupational regulatory boards evolved to understand how they work today, how we can improve their performance, and how complex relationships between the state and civil society are structured and structure board interactions. One paramount concern drives my work as a member and an analyst—protecting the public. That is the issue I always keep in the back of my mind. What protecting the public requires is rarely obvious, nor is there only one sound answer. "Protecting the public" is a complex reference frame, often ambiguous, and sometimes requiring contradictory strategies. What is the best strategy for a nonexpert member debating specialists? When should public members defer to the profession, and when should they question its assumptions? But first, we need to understand how medicine came to dominate state boards and the origin of the public voice.

Chapter 2

How Licensure Became
a Medical Institution

Eliot Freidson argues that the handful of occupations deemed to be "professions" proper have credentialed practitioners given the exclusive right to provide designated services.[1] Other social scientists provide lists of characteristics of professions or stages distinguishing emerging professions. While there is no checklist against which one can gauge an occupation's professional standing, there are features that clearly enhance a field's prestige and give its members reason to claim coveted status enjoyed by established professions like law and medicine.[2]

A body of theoretical and technical knowledge and the extensive training needed to master it mark established professional fields. Those in these fields are generally required to attend an institution of higher education and pass a licensing exam before being allowed to practice. Practitioners typically form professional organizations that establish norms governing behavior and claim the right to police themselves with minimum outside interference. To legitimize their claim as professionals, practitioners often proclaim their commitment to public service and protection of community interests. According to Harold Wilensky, "The service ideal is the pivot around which the moral claim to professional status revolves. . . . [The professional] norms dictate not only that the practitioner does technically competent, high-quality work, but that he adhere to a service ideal—devotion to the client's interests more than personal or commercial profit should guide decisions when the two are in conflict."[3] Some professions adopt formal ethical codes, but how well professionals live up to their professed ideals is open to question.[4] The debates about a trade's professional status almost invariably touch upon its members' role as guardians of common good. Professionals are eager to present themselves as faithful public servants mindful of their obligation to safeguard established values and responsive to community needs. Yet as early as 1901, Dr. T. J. Happel, secretary of the Tennessee Medical Board, wrote in the *Journal of the American Medical Society* (*JAMA*), after complaining that the attorney general would not prosecute board cases, "We are ready to assert that [medical laws] can not be enforced except through and by the medical profession. . . . The enforcement of medical laws interest[s] chiefly physicians, not the general public."[5]

The professionalization of medicine in the United States testifies to the central role that knowledge and the service ideal played in legitimizing the medical profession at the end of the nineteenth century. Yet as the following discussion shows, the major players in the professionalization process—doctors, patients, legislators, judges, investigative journalists, community activists—routinely disagree on what the public interest is, which style of medicine or standards of practice it favors, and how one should go about safeguarding communal values. Even before the American Revolution, some doctors hailed licensure as a way to improve the quality of medical care. Others staunchly opposed licensing on grounds that it limits the public's right to choose among health-care providers. And the public was split on the merits.

Many doctors espoused the belief that the public was in no position to judge its own interests, which standards of care were right, or how to enforce ethical standards. As late as 1968 Dr. Milford Rouse, an American Medical Association (AMA) president, opined that the "public recognizes it does not have the knowledge or other qualifications to evaluate medical education, medical practice, or medical competence. The public has of necessity been forced to put its trust in physicians to insure that physicians practice competently and ethically."[6] In other words, the public good is so precious and the issues of medical standards, professional misconduct, and disciplining wayward doctors are so complicated that the public should defer to professionals and stay out of the deliberations. Licensure permitted occupational market closure and also permitted the medical profession to decide the public interest.

The following historical overview centers on licensure as a focal point in the professionalization of medicine and the rhetoric of public good that various factions involved in the process invoked to justify their agendas. It should be noted that the reasons behind the licensure movement are complex, that commentators disagree about its origins and outcomes, and that even its contribution to the prestige of the medical field is open to question. One popular narrative starts with the premise that physicians are selfless professionals determined to obtain the best possible education to provide superior treatment to patients, and it is this commitment to self-improvement and quality control that lead medical professionals to clamor for licensing. This perspective puts a premium on expertise, certified knowledge, and public service, and casts licensing as an early step on the road toward professionalization.[7]

More skeptical commentators find this story self-serving. They point out that well-established physicians were those who pushed for licensure, their lofty rhetoric often obscuring a desire to limit competition and reap financial benefits by closing the market.[8] The nineteenth century witnessed the internecine warfare between medical factions of mainstream medicine, commonly referred to as "regulars" (also known as "allopaths") and "irregulars" (also known as "sects"),[9] which favored other medical systems like homeopathy or Thomsonianism (discussed below). In 1847 the regulars organized the AMA, which pushed state licensure, but it was the state medical societies who enlisted the "irregulars" in licensing drives to broaden the coalition. This was a marriage of convenience, which is why the coalition proved short lived: once the licensing movement began to bear fruit, the regulars sought to marginalize sect medical schools, casting them as inferior institutions and eventually succeeding in closing most competing training centers. The licensing movement favored one style of medicine over the other, and, as such, it threatened to close the market before substantial evidence had been accumulated to back up any medical model's claim to superior outcomes. In practice, the regulars often had as poor outcomes as other forms of medicine in the nineteenth century. Theorists favoring this perspective view the licensure movement not as a march toward better care but as a move to corner the market by the regulars who managed to dupe the politicians into legislating medical license requirements.

A third, less cynical narrative does not cast legislatures as mindless conduits for medical practitioners, focusing instead on large-scale businesses that began to dominate the marketplace. According to Paul Starr, independent practitioners clamoring for licensure needed protection in the face of the growing encroachment of big business. Licensure, in this theory, was a means of safeguarding the interests of small businesses.[10]

Licensure made headway in health-related, person-oriented occupations before business occupations.[11] Medicine may not have been well organized, but the regulars recognized the power of the sects and tried to co-opt its members into the licensure movement. Meanwhile, advancements in the field of medicine and improvements in sanitation independently contributed to the recognition of health as a public issue and reinforced the argument for licensing medical professionals.

Free Market of Medical Services

At first, the public was unsure about the wisdom of licensure. Many patients felt uneasy about the drive to license health-care practitioners, suspecting its proponents of covertly seeking to close the marketplace in medicine. From the public standpoint, anyone could sell services as a healer, just as anybody could choose his or her doctors, whatever their approach. All manners of treatment proliferated in the eighteenth and through much of the nineteenth centuries. Self-treatment was one popular option championed by the Thomsonians; homeopathy with its emphasis on nonintrusive therapies was another; the Eclectic practices were in demand as well, with their proponents railing against orthodoxies of any stripe and insisting on the right to employ practices from any model. Many of the nineteenth-century therapies, especially the interventions used by the regulars, were often worse than useless, saddling the patients with complications and adverse outcomes.[12] Until the mid-nineteenth century, the regulars relied on now-discredited practices such as bleeding, purging, and blistering to counter bad humors and stimulate nerves and muscles. The 1863 decision to ban purgatives in army hospitals provoked a strong reaction from the allopaths, who vouched for their effectiveness.[13] Dangerous practices remained in use throughout the nineteenth century even after the evidence accumulated that physicians should assist nature rather than strong-arm it. Accustomed to drastic measures, patients demanded dramatic treatments; therapies with flare drew notice.[14]

Irregular medicine had a sizable following throughout the nineteenth century, with each strain espousing its own theory of disease and often setting up training centers. Some types of medicine evolved stronger institutions than others, but each had its followers among doctors and patients. Thomsonianism, founded by Samuel Thomson (1769–1843), endorsed an egalitarian ethos that encouraged people to treat themselves, an important approach for a public that lacked access to medical care benefits and needed the Thomsonian style of medicine and self-help manuals. In 1822 Thomson published *New Guide to Health*, and by 1839 he boasted that 100,000 copies had been sold. Thomson's followers later organized medical schools.[15] Thomsonianism gained strong support in rural areas, where it was particularly influential between 1830 and 1850.

Some styles of medicine survived longer than others. Dr. Samuel Hahnemann, the creator of homeopathic medicine, had a tangible presence in the United States and Europe. A well-trained physician who believed in the importance of exercise, diet, and fresh air, he decried the bloodletting and drugging of patients favored by allopaths, urging instead small dosages of medicines and treatments aimed to alleviate the symptoms. In 1835, to shore up their influence, Hahnemann's disciples established medical schools. Although today some of the schools established as homoeopathic in the United States teach allopathic medicine, Hahnemann's perspective on medication persists into the present.[16]

Denouncing the regulars at first, Eclectics eventually joined them. Although the Eclectics had permitted women in their schools in the nineteenth century, they also joined regulars in excluding women at the end of the nineteenth century and scorned physicians who adhered to competing traditions.[17]

During the eighteenth and for much of the nineteenth century, many Americans treated themselves and had little use or money for doctors. In the eighteenth century people believed they were competent to treat illness by using common sense, reason, and books touting self-treatment. Among the books that sold well were John Tennent's *Every Man His Own Doctor; or, The Poor Planter's Physician*, Tissot's *Advice to the People in General, with Regard to their Health*, and John Theobold's *Every Man His Own Physician*.[18] Almanacs and newspapers carried stories and information about health matters. John C. Gunn's *Domestic medicine, or poor man's friend* became available in 1830, its author billing it as a complete guide for practicing medicine and surgery. The book included a complete description of an amputation and expounded on the necessity of having a sufficient number of people present to hold the patient down before beginning the operation.[19]

In the nineteenth century more physicians were available along the East Coast, but self-help maintained its appeal among those residing in other parts of the country, as well as among the financially strapped. John Oldmixon (a layman from Virginia), writing in *The British Empire in America*, maintained that Virginians "have but few doctors among them, and reckon it among their Blessings."[20] Newspapers were quick to publish stories about adverse medical outcomes and showcase disgruntled patients. Stories about the sexual exploits of doctors made the press, intriguing the public and prejudicing it against doctors. In North Carolina a tale about a medical practitioner/minister who poisoned a man in order to sleep with his wife made a stir. One physician sued a man for saying that the physician impregnated a slave.[21] Some doctors made money, but many had trouble collecting fees, and not a few were forced to abandon their practice.[22] Meanwhile, the public blamed physicians for caring more about monetary compensation than patients' health. There were charges that those who proposed restrictions did so "ostensibly for the protection of the sick, and the encouragement of medical science, but in truth, for the pecuniary benefit of a few aspiring physicians."[23] In 1833 the *New York*

Evening Star inveighed against the medical profession: "We should at once explode the whole machinery of mystification and concealment—wigs, gold canes, and the gibberish of prescriptions—which serves but as a cloak to ignorance and legalized murder."[24] Members of the public did not hesitate to pass judgment on the quality of medical care, with few patients considering health care a public issue requiring state involvement. One positive reaction, though, came during the trial of Samuel Thomson, leader of the Thomsonian self-help movement, when he was accused of murdering a patient in 1809. His trial furnished a venue for promoting his method, and the jury refused to convict him.[25]

During the second half of the eighteenth and first half of the nineteenth century, allopathic medical societies pressed their members to adopt regular medicine as the only acceptable style, though evidence was still scant as to which type of medicine was more efficacious. Allopathic doctors' efforts to pass legislation were not completely successful. Struggling for survival, medical societies positioned themselves as the establishments whose members had the exclusive right to collect fees for the practice of medicine, but many doctors found a way around that limitation by selling medicines.[26] Not accidentally, medical society members tended to come from prominent, higher-status families. Physicians without the right pedigree contented themselves with less-affluent clientele and often had to supplement their income with alternative employment. When South Carolina doctors moved in 1755 to set up a society for "the Better Support of the Dignity, the Privileges, and Emoluments of their Humane Art," they found themselves derided by critics who suggested that the society's objective was to harness patients' dollars rather than safeguard public health. A newspaper article claimed that physicians were worried about collecting their payments and having to attend patients in inclement weather. When the members of the society resolved to withhold treatment from patients who did not pay a "reasonable" fee, the local newspaper was inundated with letters from outraged patients.[27] As these examples suggest, the public was far from sure that any drive for licensure was meant to protect the common good.

What doctors saw as ways to ensure the rights of medical professionals commensurate with their contribution to community, the public tended to perceive as unseemly attempts to protect special interests. Nor was the public easily swayed by the rhetoric of protecting patients from swindlers and con artists. The Medical Society of New Jersey announced in its inaugural statement that it aimed to discourage "quacks, mountebanks, imposters or other ignorant pretenders of medicine,"[28] but as medical historian Richard Shryock points out, doctors wrote such articles to promote licensure and scare the public. A man believed to be a member of the Boston medical society, formed in the 1730s, wrote an article in the *Boston Weekly Newsletter* in response to an epidemic of diphtheria and scarlet fever: "Methinks it would be . . . of no great Difficulty to concert some proper measures for regulating the Practice of Physick throughout this Province . . . so that no person shall be allowed to practice Physick within . . . this Province, unless he be first examined by such regular, approved . . . Physicians and Surgeons as the Honourable Court shall see meet to appoint."[29] The author went on to say that if a doctor did not pass the examination, the patient should be treated by a nurse, a safer alternative. In 1803 the Medical Society of Massachusetts granted only seventy doctors admission out of a larger pool of applicants, but few privileges could be gained from society membership: library use, lecture attendance, and meeting participation. Even in this uncertain environment, the sects continued to flourish, as patients sought all manner of health-care practitioners.

The competition among different models of medicine was fierce, as was the competition between the schools and proponents of licensure. Medical societies policed their members' contacts with nonmembers.[30] Medical schools provided strong opposition to the societies' efforts to license physicians, deeming medical degrees as sufficient for practicing medicine. At the onset of the nineteenth century, four medical schools trained physicians in the United States. The number grew to 187 by 1904, but by 1920 only 85 remained.[31] The growth in Eclectic schools helped alleviate the shortage of doctors in rural areas, especially in the Midwest.[32] Any graduate from a chartered medical school could practice in most states, and legislatures seemed eager to grant a charter to any medical school, making critics complain that anyone looking to make a living could set up a school for training doctors.[33] Unconnected to universities or hospitals, most schools were proprietary. Students paid faculty directly; schools profited by enrolling as many students as possible for the shortest period to maximize fees collected. Little incentive existed to strengthen the requirements, for such practices increased tuition costs, discouraging enrollment. Schools competed with medical societies for control over standards, each insisting they were better positioned to safeguard standards. The competition and resulting suspicion were so great that in 1839, when the Medical Society of New York issued an invitation to all colleges and societies to attend a meeting, the organizers received no response.[34] The often rancorous conflict between the schools and the medical societies deterred licensing. To gain greater control of education and to limit the power of the schools, the newly formed (1847) American Medical Association proposed moving licensing from local medical societies to the state.[35] Major universities lengthened study, started to pay faculty salaries, and had lower enrollments before states passed modern licensing statutes.[36] In his 1883 AMA presidential address, Dr. Nathan Davis laid out a broad agenda, calling for fortifying premedical school academic requirements, lengthening mandatory training, instituting medical boards to administer licensing exams, and rallying local professional societies behind this national agenda.

The profit motive drove much of the proliferation of medical schools and impeded the licensure drive. Patient needs played a peripheral role in the growth of the medical establishment and articulation of standards of care. The weeding out of medical schools would mean fewer, albeit better-trained doctors, but if many doctors were eliminated and students were scared away by high tuition fees, fewer doctors would be available to serve the less well off or those living in more isolated areas. The critical public issue—access to health care—remained unarticulated and unexplored.

The AMA pressed hard on the issue of insufficient training. Dr. Perry Millard, vice president of the AMA and member of the Medical Society of Michigan, wrote in 1887 that "it seems quite absurd that the propriety of regulating the practice of medicine should be questioned . . . the only opposition . . . comes principally from the representatives of the seventy-nine medical schools of the United States. . . . It is certainly the duty of the chosen representatives of the people, the legislature, to protect an ignorant and credulous public."[37] Some thought licensing by the states would resolve educational issues. In Millard's view, not only should state boards create minimum standards, but the "Respective Boards should be empowered to revoke licenses for chronic inebriety and grossly dishonorable conduct. The power to refuse or revoke a license should only be used in flagrant cases." The boards were supposed to be appointed by the governor, confirmed in the senate, and "aim to obtain the most intelligent and honorable gentlemen at his command."[38] Issues of character and physician's standing in the community grew in importance toward the end of the nineteenth century, hinting at a stake the public had in licensing outcomes.

Legislatures, not doctors, were behind some early efforts to promote labor regulation of doctors.[39] These laws generally were not enforced. Virginia passed a law in 1639 making it possible to arrest physicians who charged unreasonable fees and sanction physicians who neglected patients or failed to help persons in medical need, but little evidence of enforcement exists. In 1736 the legislature enacted a law that established fees, distinguished the amount that could be charged between "in town" and "out of town" visits, and stipulated that university-trained physicians could charge twice the fees permitted others, but it let the law lapse after two years.[40] The provincial assembly in

New York passed a licensing law in 1760 requiring all physicians to be examined by government officials assisted by reputable physicians.[41] Again, little evidence exists of its enforcement. Connecticut newspapers pronounced their medical society monopolistic, which thwarted further legislative action. Medical societies continued to push for laws restricting competition. In 1818 the Massachusetts Medical Society convinced the legislature to enact a law that only those licensed by the medical society or a graduate of Harvard College could recover debts.[42] Weaned on the notions of egalitarianism and unrestricted trade, the public frowned on the prospect of creating a state-supported niche for an occupation, opting instead for the right to choose.

Clearly common good was implicated, but what that was remained hotly contested. For example, in the first half of the nineteenth century, legislators often enacted licensure statutes only to rescind them under public pressure within a few years because of conflicts within the profession as well as popular demand.[43] New York, the first state to try to develop standards in 1760, vacated all pertinent laws in 1844. Illinois implemented licensure in 1817, modified it in 1825, and repealed it in 1826. Ohio first licensed physicians in 1811 and repealed the law in 1833. South Carolina abolished all penalties for practicing without a license. In some states the medical societies had the power to license, but in others, the power resided with the state government. Using the language of public protection, the court supported licensing by the medical societies as other avenues into the profession were possible, and the law was intended only to advise. Chief Justice Lemuel Shaw of Massachusetts wrote in 1835: "It appears to us that the leading and sole purpose of this act was to guard the public against ignorance, negligence, and carelessness in the members of one of the most useful professions."[44] The market remained largely unrestricted, and by 1845 ten states had repealed licensure, while eight states had never enacted them.[45]

Sanitation and Improvements in Medical Knowledge

Before the public and the state could be convinced of their stake in healthcare issues, they had to be convinced that medicine produced health and that, consequently, health was a public issue. To achieve their goal, the proponents of licensing had to frame their concern as a public health matter. Heightened attention to urban sanitation and water treatment played a role in educating the public about its stake in the ongoing debate.[46]

By the mid-nineteenth century, physicians, engineers, and citizens banded together to eliminate contagious diseases.[47] Women physicians played a prominent role in these groups.[48] Lay members sat on executive committees of public health organizations with local officials.[49] If public participation was possible, Barbara Rosenkrantz insists, it was because many of the physicians involved in the movement understood public health as civic duty rather than as a professional responsibility. As the century came to a close, such groups were reconstituted, with physicians in the majority as providers of "rational and scientific" services.[50] Public members often remained prominent in such organizations throughout the Progressive era.[51] But the bioscientific terms used in public health board discourses underscored that the issues would ultimately be framed as medical. Once public health hazards were cast as medical problems, public participation seemed increasingly meddlesome to professionals.[52]

As it became clear that sanitation and clean water affected everyone, the media focused on these issues, attracting readership among the general public.[53] Progressive era politics sensitized the public to the notion, powerfully articulated by John Dewey, that "exercise of the profession has consequences so wide-spread that the examination and licensing of persons who practice them becomes a public matter."[54] With the public weighing in on the issues of where to build roads, whether to start new school buildings, and how to care for the elderly, poor, and sick, the need to protect the public interest became more apparent. In this climate, legislators and judges began to warm up to the notion that licensure statutes had merit and required enforcement.

Licensure received a further boost from major advances in medicine in the second half of the nineteenth century. New discoveries were so impressive that some irregulars hastened to join the regulars, who in turn endorsed some homeopathic ideas, such as the need to moderate heroic treatments. Innovations made longer courses of education necessary and encouraged Americans to train in Europe.[55] Nevertheless, new knowledge and treatment techniques spread slowly in the United States.

Understanding the importance of diagnostic tools increased after 1860. An 1866 article by Dr. Eduoard Seguin featured the discussion of the ophthalmoscope, laryngoscope, binaural stethoscope, and clinical thermometer.[56] Henry Bigelow described his successful removal of large tumors in 1846. It took longer for germ theory, developed in midcentury Europe, to make inroads in the United States. A major textbook did not mention it until its 1881 edition. According to John Duffy, the public had a greater interest in germ theory than physicians.[57] Dr. John Erichsen, a British physician visiting the United States in 1874, expressed concern about medical education, especially the failure to use antiseptics, which had been developed in 1867.[58] Dr. Robert Weir sounded a similar alarm when speaking to the New York Medical Society three years later.[59] While anesthesia quickly caught on for surgery, the use of antiseptics took longer to gain acceptance, despite high death rates from surgery unaided by antiseptic treatment. The first antiseptic surgery in the United States took place in Boston twelve years after Dr. Joseph Lister told the British Medical Association that his wards were free of sepsis after nine months of using antiseptics. The doctors attending President James Garfield when he was shot in 1881 did not use antiseptics, but by 1885 major urban hospitals employed them fairly consistently.[60] Those developments gathered speed as states passed licensure statutes.[61]

The AMA still needed a strategy for advancing licensure in the face of strong opposition from those who practiced "irregular" medicine and from schools. Improvements in medical education and the spread of new knowledge and techniques benefited some doctors and some of the public. Most bills reaching state legislatures included several pathways for practice, effectively allowing all varieties of medical practice and weakening internal opposition. An essential element for the successful passing of licensure statutes was recasting health as a public issue.

Licensure Debates Heat Up

Reducing economic competition in the medical field promised to strengthen its prestige by making the profession more exclusive and educated.[62] Dr. Perry Millard in 1887 claimed that the rate of increase in the number of physicians was 5 percent, while the population grew only 2 percent. Moreover, the ratio of doctors per person was at least twice as high in the United States as in Europe: "It is, however, ordained that in our profession, the noblest of them all, we shall be left to a competition that is intolerable to an educated man. . . . [The] United States is the only civilized country that is devoid of restrictions regulating the practice of medicine."[63] Improvements in education, while potentially beneficial to patients, were also understood to enhance the profession's standing in the community. In his 1846 speech before the New York Medical and Surgical Society, Dr. F. Campbell Stewart expressed his concern about low educational standards: "I am bound to acknowledge that, in science at least, the profession in this country is far behind the medical community in other countries . . . owing to the wrong and faulty system of medical education."[64] Status was on his mind as well; "It is most humiliating to us to know that none of our colleges are recognized by European schools as on a footing of full equality."[65]

In the mid-nineteenth century, regulation in the United States was limited largely to oversight of railroads, but state regulation expanded rapidly to health-related occupations in the last quarter of the nineteenth century.[66]

Public opinion and scholarly debate provided little support for the restrictions on medical practice imposed by licensure. Social Darwinists opposed licensing on the ground that all regulations are harmful. If the public could not understand who was a safe practitioner and died as a result, then the population stock would only improve. Herbert Spencer argued that ignorance was not an excuse for regulation.[67] William James, a pragmatist philosopher and graduate of the Harvard medical school, argued against regulation for different reasons. When the physicians in Massachusetts wanted to require all "faith curers" or "mind curers" to hold medical degrees, he protested in the *Boston Evening Transcript*: "But their facts are patent and startling and anything that interferes with the multiplication of such facts, and from our freest opportunity of observing and studying them, will, I believe, be a public calamity. The law now proposed will so interfere, simply because mind-curers will not take the examinations."[68] The bill was tabled for four years; when it resurfaced in 1898, James testified against the bill, accusing the medical profession of "the fiercely partisan attitude of a powerful trade union, demanding legislation against the competition of the 'scabs.'"[69]

Some organized to resist licensing. The National Constitutional Liberty League, founded in Boston in the 1890s, lobbied against requirements and distributed literature quoting William Gladstone and Thomas Henry Huxley, who supported the *caveat emptor* tradition. Mark Twain concurred on the ground that it was his own body and, hence, his own harm.[70] The editors of the Wisconsin press opposed including advertising by doctors as unprofessional conduct in the first revision of the 1897 practice act, as newspapers feared a loss of advertising revenue from physicians.[71]

Many observers of early boards—including the British playwright George Bernard Shaw, who wrote a series of articles in the 1920s and 1930s—condemned the British medical regulatory system.[72] Louis Caldwell argued in a 1923 law review article that, "as a rule, when there has been public sentiment at all on questions of such acts, it has not been on the side of the regular physicians."[73] He insisted further that medical boards were captives of the profession and characterized licensing as "protection against competition."[74] Many commentators favored choice and felt partial to alternative health-care methods such as patent medicines, a big business.[75] When doctors were brought to trial for practicing without a license or even a degree, juries would sometimes refuse to sanction. In a rural Louisiana 1894 case, one Dr. Allen, who had neither a license to practice nor a medical degree, was indicted by a grand jury, but when he said that he would give up the practice, the jury withdrew the indictment. Dr. Allen continued to practice until 1920.[76] But the public lacked political clout and was not sufficiently organized to stop licensure, and once legislatures and courts invoked the common good as a reason to support licensing, public opposition quieted.

Affirming the right to license and exclude unlicensed physicians from medical practice was a local act involving local players and requiring local campaigns. Although the practice of medicine remained "in a state of confusion," many elite doctors were using new life-saving techniques.[77] Most state medical societies agreed to license all practicing doctors, which prevented the medical community splitting along sectarian lines. Medicine was among the first occupations to gain licensure, but dentists and pharmacists claimed even greater success in establishing licensing requirements.[78] "Licensing, rather than being identified with power and privilege, as it had been in the 1830s, became part of the resistance of a threatened petite bourgeoisie."[79] The fact that legislatures first granted licensure to occupations concerned with health and cleanliness confirms a vital link between the successes of licensure and the public health movement.

Nevertheless, it was the occupations themselves that pushed for licensure, though physicians were not yet particularly well organized. Strong state societies were still a rarity, and it was only after 1903, when the AMA finally removed most of its objections to homeopaths and Eclectics, that the medical societies made strides toward increasing licensing requirements.[80] By the turn of the twentieth century, most states had passed licensure statutes.[81]

Licensure statutes supported different schools of medicine and alternative pathways to licensure. In the mid-1870s Louisiana and Michigan physicians set up licensing boards uniting regulars and homeopaths. In Massachusetts, the regulars and the Eclectics were part of the same examining board. In Tennessee several groups joined forces to form the first licensing board in 1889.[82] Many regulars continued to frown on alternative approaches but included their practitioners in the licensing laws for the sake of licensing.[83] Pathways to licensure included a diploma, an exam, or some years in local practice.[84] The acceptance of regular medicine practice by many of the irregulars contributed to rapid enactment of the medical practice acts mostly between 1855 (in Indiana) and 1896 (in California).[85] Rhode Island provides an example of a late licensing statute (1895) where the avenues for licensure included a diploma from a legally chartered medical school in "good standing," marked by length of study, clinical instruction, regular attendance, and required exams, good facilities for instruction, clinics and dissections; or examination by the board; or practice of medicine in Rhode Island before January 1, 1892.[86] Most applicants had substantial training. Of the first 350 applicants, 211 claimed four or more years of medical school, and most had more than three.[87] Many described additional apprenticeships, internships, or study in Europe. Two hundred eighty-nine listed their practices as "regular" or "allopathic," forty-one claimed homeopathy, three identified as "Eclectic," and seventeen gave mixed or unique responses.[88] Most, but not all, received their training in well-established medical schools. One applicant sent a handwritten letter to the board about the disappearance of his school: "Your fear of the 3rd is justified. The College . . . Charted in N.Y. located 6th Av. New York City—at the time I graduated. Dr. Thall died fifteen years ago and the locality was changed, where I do not know."[89] Only fourteen of the applicants were women.[90] The strength of the sects had waned before the licensure movement began to bear fruit, with many irregulars adopting the treatments of the regulars.[91] The AMA code of ethics prohibited consultation with irregulars, but almost half the states had sect representation on their licensure boards (twenty-three states). The practice of medicine was becoming more standardized, and doctors studied longer.[92]

Public protection was not high on the AMA agenda. We can glean that from the vigor with which the organization worked to block malpractice suits and to institute bans on doctors testifying against each another. In 1887 the Michigan state medical society voted to prohibit its members from testifying voluntarily against each other.[93] By 1910 the medical societies in thirteen states offered legal help to physicians facing malpractice suits. When Dr. J. E. Stubbs addressed the Physicians Club of Chicago in 1899, he argued it was in the best interests of the profession to conceal medical errors from the public. Dr. Joseph McCormack urged Kentucky physicians never to disparage each other; he thought that licensing laws and increased educational require-ments would reduce the number of incompetent doctors and make malpractice suits rare.[94]

With the onset of the Progressive era, it was common for physicians to mention patients as main beneficiaries of the licensure policies advanced by medical societies. When the North Carolina state medical association reinsti-tuted itself in 1849, it highlighted its new mission as promoting "all measures of a professional nature that are adaptable to the relief of suffering humanity, and to improve the health and protect the lives of the community." However, this reference to common good could hardly obscure the organization's goal to delegitimize the irregulars on the pretext that "our titles are assumed and our privileges claimed by charlatans of every caste."[95] Anxieties about doctors' professional standing remained high. Dr. F. Campbell Stewart aired them while addressing the New York Medical and Surgical Society: "That there is a great want of respect and regard for what is called the regular profession, is

I think, abundantly manifested by the unconcealed and open efforts to injure it, as evinced both by the encouragement of quackery . . . and by a constant endeavor to find fault with, condemn, and ridicule the art and those who practice it."[96] The drive to improve medical training and institute licensure often appeared to have more to do with the economic benefits and status needs of the medical profession than public good.

Judges supported licensure on the theory that the public was unable to distinguish high-from poor-quality medical care and their perception of health as a public good. Lawyers were self-regulating.[97] Judges used the language of expertise and public health to justify their holdings. In *Dent v. West Virginia* (1889), the U.S. Supreme Court confirmed the right to license physicians based on the expertise necessary to assess the skills of those claiming to be physicians and the potential consequences of incorrect assessments.[98] Marmaduke Dent, a graduate of the American Medical Eclectic College of Cincinnati, continued to practice after he was denied a license in West Virginia. He was convicted and fined under a West Virginia 1882 statute that declared a physician had to graduate from a reputable medical school, or had practiced medicine for ten years in the state, or had passed an exam to be licensed. Dent had practiced for six years, meeting none of the criteria.

Justice Stephen Field, known as a protector of individual rights against state interference, made a case that no one had the right to practice a profession without the minimum qualifications and that only an "authority competent to judge" could determine whether the criteria had been met. The justice's opinion placed that authority in the hands of the profession on the grounds that medical licensing was a public health matter and that the state had broad powers to protect citizens lacking in the knowledge needed to guard their interests. The courts further affirmed that boards could and should assess physicians' moral character. In *Hawker v. New York* (1898), the Supreme Court upheld a law barring convicted felons from practicing medicine, stating that bad character was a sufficient basis to deny a license because of the right of the state to protect the health of the public.[99] Hawker was convicted of a felony, upheld in 1878, for performing an abortion. After serving time in jail, he resumed the practice of medicine. Despite the fact that his felony conviction was prior to the new law making it illegal to practice with a felony conviction, the Supreme Court ruled that in order to protect the public, good character was more important than the matter of timing of the law.

Although regulation would continue to come under attack by the Supreme Court, medical licensing since *Dent* had been upheld by the courts on account of its impact on public health.[100] In 1905, Justice Rufus Peckham argued that working in a bakery for long hours did not interfere with the public health as existing restrictions enforced the cleanliness (health) of bakeries.[101] Soon afterwards in *Watson v. Maryland* (1910), the Supreme Court affirmed that the police power of the state extended to occupations connected with public health and that it was reasonable that a physician should be required to register to practice medicine.[102] Self-regulation was another issue that came to prominence as the drive to licensure began to bear fruit. Once their claim to exclusive expertise and high moral character was accepted, physicians felt emboldened to assert their right to self-regulate.[103]

Self-Regulation as a Pinnacle of Professional Power

The medical profession worked hard to assert its right to require licensing exams and to close "substandard" medical schools, its effort aided by a private foundation. In 1925 the AMA printed a book by a lawyer, Mr. Harry Kelly, on medical regulation, in which he first makes a statement about the good physicians do for society: "The physician's occupation has become probably the world's greatest profession; . . . great in the priceless knowledge, skill and services supplied by them to relieve suffering."[104] But the purpose of licensing is not to restrict competition, we are told: "It will not escape the notice of the most casual observer that the best qualified physician, instead of being injured by competition from the ill prepared doctor, is more likely to be enriched by repairing the injuries."[105] The need for self-regulation arises from the profession's scientific background as well as from the complex morality of doctoring: "But the layman's unaided estimate of a physician is more likely to be wrong than right. . . . Determining whether a physician is competent to practice his profession involves appraisement of the physician's understanding of matters of science with which most persons are unfamiliar. Determination of a physician's moral character is a task in which persons of the widest experience with are not so sure of their judgment as to refuse the assistance of those who have made an actual investigation and ascertained the facts about the particular man."[106] The average person is cast here as something of a dupe, an image consistent with the first code of medical ethics that played up the physicians' credentials as guardians of common good and scientific knowledge, downplaying the public's ability to fend for itself.[107] Laypersons were perceived as incompetent. The ability of experts to self-regulate was held in the highest regard by the profession, taking for granted doctors would use their technical knowledge to make decisions consistent with and beneficial to the collective good. In 1927 a critical Dewey wrote: "For most men, save the scientific workers, science is a mystery in the hands of initiates, who have become adept in virtue of following ritualistic ceremonies from which the profane herd is excluded."[108] The premise that medical expertise alone should define professional practices makes doctors' actions immune to challenge by nonexperts.[109]

Many social scientists accepted the profession's claim that lack of expertise makes it difficult for the public to render judgment on their best interests and that professional codes of conduct are sufficient to keep doctors in line.[110] Self-regulation seemed logical,[111] indeed inevitable.[112] According to the prevailing belief, medical students learn to act ethically in the course of training, which teaches them that altruism is good for business.[113] Board supervision would ensure that the professional standards were maintained. A strong professional community could police itself.

Even in that era, some public intellectuals saw a different side to a strong professional community. Dewey wrote, "A class of experts is inevitably so removed from common interests as to become a class with private interests and private knowledge, which in social matters is not knowledge at all."[114] But such warnings remained unheeded by a poorly organized public. The licensure movement contributed to the creation of a powerful medical community with a self-justificatory discourse, organizations to meet its needs, ethical codes, and training institutions for its members. Interacting largely within that community, doctors identified with and developed bonds with the profession, which further facilitated recognition of their collective interests.[115]

The Medical Profession Develops a Community of Interest

The medical practice acts that created licensure provided new opportunities for social closure.[116] Licensing board activities strengthened the sense of a community among medical professionals who increasingly adopted the rhetoric of public service to buttress their prestige.[117] Meanwhile, the public had little understanding of, and even less input into, how its interests were defined. Licensing board members were well-established professionals (typically general practitioners), almost universally male (only one female doctor served on a state board in 1968), advanced in age (average age of 58.3 years), focused primarily on writing and grading licensure exams, and firmly committed to professional autonomy and fee-for-service practice models.[118]

Having assumed the right to define the proper doctor-patient relationship, medical boards shunned publicity and kept their procedures closed to the public. Boards largely succeeded in convincing the public that doctors were altruistic in their aspirations, ethical in their conduct, and perfectly capable of ridding themselves of a few bad apples through internal oversight. State courts generally went along with the notion that professionals were fit to sort out their own affairs. When medical boards disciplined their brethren, it was not so much on account of their incompetence as on the grounds of deficient moral character. Some business practices came under attack, including those clearly beneficial to some segments of the public.

In Oklahoma the medical board and medical society waged a war against Dr. Michael A. Shadid, a graduate of the Washington University medical school, who had built a community hospital catering to the needs of poor patients who received treatment for a yearly fee.[119] In his autobiography, *A Doctor for the People,* Dr. Shadid recalled his encounters with the Oklahoma board and medical society whose members set up a blockade around his cooperative hospital. When young doctors expressed interest in joining his practice, they received this warning from the local medical society: "The community hospital is in disrepute with the medical profession of the state, the head of the institution being ineligible for membership in the county society for various reasons, several of which I would not care to put in writing."[120] In 1936 Dr. Shadid received a letter from an unknown physician who explained what was happening in the medical society:

> Now their scheme is this. . . . These proposed amendments to the Medical Practice Act have been drawn to look innocent, but they openly state it is to put your institution out of business. . . . I am reliably informed charges are to be brought before the Medical Board at the next meeting to revoke the license of you and Dr. T. This is to be done in order to hurt your influence with the Legislature, the Governor and the people. The amendments would take this law out of the hands of the governor and the State, where it rightly belongs, and put it under that political bunch, the Oklahoma State Medical Association.[121]

The new governor turned the case over to the health commissioner, a member of the medical society, who summoned Dr. Shadid to appear before the State Board of Medical Examiners on charges of advertising, fleecing the public, and "steerage" or soliciting patients. The board did not sanction him.

Medical groups worked hard to establish organizations that would strengthen licensure standards with minimum input from legislators and the public.[122] The twin objectives behind this drive were to raise licensure requirements and standardize medical training. Upholding the right of states to set their own standards, the state courts showed themselves unwilling to join the fight for national standards. The reciprocity question—the right to transfer a medical license issued in one state to a different jurisdiction—remained a thorny issue throughout the twentieth and into the twenty-first century.

The AMA managed to gain national footing in the early twentieth century by lending its support to the local medical societies and beginning to integrate state and national level organizations' agendas. The AMA also made headway with medical specialists who were reluctant to join the national organization at first.[123] In 1901, about 25 percent of the regular physicians were members of a state association, and only 9 percent joined the AMA. To improve its standing, the AMA reformed its constitution, reframing its membership as a right of licensed doctors rather than as a privilege, and permitting its members to consult with all licensed practitioners.[124] Local association members were granted automatic membership in a statewide association whose members chose their AMA representatives. This reorganization bolstered the national effort to standardize medical training requirements. The Federation of State Medical Boards (FSMB, or Federation), founded in 1912, like the AMA, enjoyed limited local influence. Independently from the AMA, state medical societies wielded great influence on state licensing boards; membership in the state medical society was often a prerequisite for physician board membership.[125]

Creating new educational standards for licensure had a major impact on the number of medical schools, which in turn affected the public good in a manner that called for close scrutiny. The National Confederation of State Examining and Licensing Boards, formed in 1891, worked to increase medical education requirements. By the end of the first quarter of the twentieth century, most states required exams for new licensees; these changes had to happen locally. A new representative voting system, instituted by the AMA in 1901, helped to achieve this goal. Between 1901 and 1907, membership in state societies doubled to 70,000, which boded well for coordinating national and state policies.[126] The exam requirements made it more difficult to obtain a license, while the ranking of medical schools led to many closings. In 1894, the Illinois State Board of Health published a list of approved medical schools, and two years later the AMA issued its first assessment of medical schools.[127] The AMA then created the Council on Medical Education, which produced annual reports on school inspections and began to certify schools.[128] Initially, the AMA furnished its evaluations exclusively to a given school and licensing board, but, beginning in 1907, *JAMA* made the exam pass rate public for each school.[129] The council became a quasi-public agency, and by 1905 it endorsed standards higher than those of the American Association of Medical Colleges (AAMC).[130]

The Illinois board and the Council on Medical Education's evaluations set the stage for the Flexner Report (1910), which was funded by the Carnegie Foundation in 1908 to evaluate medical schools. The Flexner Report aroused both the public and the legislatures, something that the profession alone did not achieve.[131] Only Johns Hopkins, Harvard, and Case Western medical schools received very high marks. About half of all schools received poor evaluations and either merged or went out of existence between 1904 and 1920.[132] The elimination of schools generated controversy within the profession, but it died down as physicians realized that, with fewer physicians, the demand for their services was bound to rise. By raising standards, medical organizations managed to lower the number of new physicians, thus ensuring their financial interests and reassuring the public of its safety. Yet the increased standards meant not only increased safety—it also signified diminishing access to medical care. According to Dr. Robert Derbyshire of the Federation, "The AMA, aided by certain foundations and supported by state boards, achieved both its goals by this decade; that is, an improvement in the selection and education of doctors, and a reduction in the ratio of doctors to population."[133] Richard Shryock, a historian, thought that with the closing of many poor medical schools by 1920 the "safe general practitioner at last began to emerge."[134] Others sounded the alarm because schools that admitted women, blacks, and nonallopathic practitioners were among those that fared worst in the new ranking system and, thus, faced closure.[135]

The AMA asked state medical societies to appoint licensing board members who would support reforms in educational standards, and most states did just that. But local medical boards reserved the right to produce their own exams.[136] The goal of national standardization remained elusive. There was little national associations could do besides trying to persuade local societies and boards to streamline policies or standards. The American Confederation of Reciprocating, Examining, and Licensing Boards, established in 1902 to encourage interstate acceptance of licenses, joined forces with the National Confederation of Licensing Boards in 1912 to form the Federation of State Medical Boards. Nevertheless, the FSMB had no coercive power over state boards. A new organization established in 1915, the National Board of Medical Examiners (NBME), was necessary to create a national exam that would help further standardization of medical education and allow greater reciprocity among the states. The development and use of a national exam required cooperation among national organizations and the willingness of state medical societies to encourage boards to adopt it. Nevertheless, many states required or accepted local state developed exams through the 1960s.

The major drive toward a national licensing exam goes back to 1902 when the AMA called for one in *JAMA*.[137] One editorial claimed at the time that "it won't happen because of the multiplicity of boards of examiners, the majority of which are created by political influence and not by the selection of members qualified for the positions of examiners in scientific medicine."[138] In April 1915 the FSMB produced the first volume of the *Federation Bulletin* that lamented the lack of uniformity in state licensing laws. This topic figured prominently at the first Federation meeting and many that followed.[139] The formation of NBME testified to the organizers' improved political skills. The AMA president, Dr. William Rodman, announced its 1915 formation financed by the Carnegie Foundation. Dr. Walter Bierring of FSMB was one of its chief supporters. Still, many others feared the move as a step toward national licensure. In 1916 the AMA delegates voted to accept the report of its Council on Medical Education in support of the NBME. The NBME board brought together all the interested groups: board members came from the federal government (six), the FSMB (one), the AAMC (one), the American College of Surgeons (one), the AMA (three), and three members at large.[140] A close alliance between the Federation and the NBME was formed in part because Dr. Bierring served not only as secretary to the FSMB but also as an NBME board member and president.[141]

Designed to facilitate reciprocity, the new national exam did not immediately produce the intended results. Initially, only eight states accepted the exam, first given in 1916. By 1949, forty-five states endorsed it.[142] Despite its acceptance in most states, only 25 percent of American medical school graduates took it in 1940; the majority opted for state examinations. The Federation had some influence over state boards but not enough to effect the change. When the NBME introduced a new objective exam in 1953, ten states that had accepted the exam made an about-face and refused to endorse the results. Some states required additional local exams, and a handful maintained state exams as late as 1964.[143] In several jurisdictions, higher passing scores were required than others, and foreign-trained physicians were barred from taking the state exams. All such policies led to fewer doctors practicing in a given state, thereby increasing the economic prospects and social cachet of the licensed physicians.[144] In 1935, seven states had policies in place that assured that no foreign-trained physician could be licensed in the state. The NBME further disenfranchised foreign-trained physicians by denying them the right to take its exam after 1952.

When the NBME stopped examining foreign graduates, the Federation counteracted by developing the FLEX exam, which reopened the door to foreign medical school graduates wishing to practice in the United States.[145] Nine hundred applicants took the FLEX exam when first offered in 1968, yet only seven states recognized the results. By 1972, forty-two states accepted the exam, and in 1979 Florida, the last state to do so, accepted it as well. Differences in exams and scoring procedures continued to be a thorny issue: "Many boards of Medical examiners are in ill repute with both the public and legislatures. They are accused, sometimes unjustly, of fostering monopolies and keeping competition out. In at least two states this criticism is more justified as board members freely admit that their examinations are designed not so much to test the knowledge of applicants for licensure but to keep the number of physicians at a level optimal to the establishment."[146] One clear benefit of the FLEX exam was the sizable revenue the examination fees produced for the Federation, weakening its financial relationship with the AMA, which had funded the *Federation Bulletin* and FSMB meetings.

Backed by local medical societies, licensing boards wielded considerable power. The Federation's authority did not extend beyond its mandate to recommend board organization and exams. State boards retained close ties with medical societies as many governors in 1969 still had to appoint board members from lists provided by the state medical societies. In two states the members were picked directly by the medical societies, and in one case the board was a committee chosen from medical society membership. Derbyshire, president of the FSMB, wrote in 1965, "It is strange that the medical societies can exercise so much influence in the appointment.... They [medical societies] claim to have removed politics from the board.... [The medical societies] ignore professional and educational attributes, endorsing some faithful political stalwart."[147] Patient access to board activities was not considered, largely on the grounds that exam standards and training were sufficient to ensure quality control.

Licensure suggested policing of problem doctors, but in practice few were reported to the boards for misconduct of any sort. This was hardly a surprise given that medical professionals were deterred by professional codes from reporting problem colleagues, while the public was deemed incompetent to judge what constituted good medical care and knew nothing of boards, anyway. The few disciplinary cases there were entailed moral or ethical issues. Derbyshire found 938 licensure actions nationally from 1963 to 1967, of which 334 resulted in revocation, 375 in probation, 161 in suspension, and 68 in reprimands. Almost half involved narcotics violations (440), and 41 entailed accusations of alcoholism. Felony convictions (72) and abortions (71) followed mental incompetence (94) and fraud (74). There was no category for incompetence in the practice of medicine, and only seven doctors were sanctioned for gross malpractice in four years.[148] Earlier in a 1916 Rhode Island case a young female patient died from what the newspaper called a "criminal operation," likely an abortion.[149] The physician was tried in court and found guilty. In another case, the Rhode Island board declined to revoke a doctor's license after a finding of guilt for distributing drugs in violation of the Harrison Narcotics Act in federal court (May 2, 1919). On December 9, 1920, the physician appeared before the Rhode Island State Board of Health to answer the charge of unprofessional conduct resulting from the conviction. "At this meeting the charges were not sustained and were dismissed."[150]

The medical profession's ethics did little to protect the public; boards punished physicians for testifying against other doctors. For nine years the Arizona board refused to license a doctor who had helped the Illinois attorney general locate problem practitioners. He had incurred the ire of doctors in Illinois who contacted the Arizona board when he moved there. Arizona denied him a license based on his unfitness to practice medicine despite having a letter from the Illinois attorney general explaining why doctors wrote letters to destroy his career. The court finally saw the political nature of licensure denial and restored the practitioner's standing in 1960.[151] It is questionable whether public good entered the first decision.

Boards rarely mentioned public protection. The Federation's first Model Act (1957) included such language; few used it. For its part, the public neither appeared overly concerned about the boards' activities, nor did it have any voice in the matter. Although most citizens had little idea about the medical board practices, the press recognized health as a public issue from the inception of boards.[152] On July 14, 1913, the *New York Times* reported, "Recognition of the fact that the treatment of disease is a public, rather than a private concern is becoming steadily clearer, day by day, and the Federation's privilege will be to emphasize and extend this truth."[153] Meanwhile, boards continued to function as medical organizations catering to their constituency of physicians, while state courts made narrow decisions after cases such as *Dent* and *Hawker* and showed little sign of factoring public interest into their decisions.

Criticism from Within and Outside

As the above discussion suggests, medical boards helped frame economic and moral issues as medical rather than public concerns. The profession prided itself on having the expertise and the moral standing to determine what the public needed. The profession did an effective job of developing organizations to promote its social closure, continuing to insulate themselves from the public. While the profession raised medical standards in the name of public interest, it controlled the number of practitioners and worked against insurance plans. Patients able to pay for health care saw standards of care improve. That was not the case with patients of limited means, who often faced the loss of access to medical care, or those damaged by incompetence or negligence. The public interest in access to care remained largely unaddressed. But in 1943 the Supreme Court rejected the AMA's push to prohibit group practice of medicine.[154] The state stepped in.

By midcentury, the state and the public saw cracks in the health-care system, and the broader culture became critical of experts. The notion that doctors were fully capable of policing themselves came under attack. Because doctors restricted the scope of practice of other health-care professionals and discouraged the reporting of possible physician misconduct, other actors had to be brought into the oversight process. If the medical field lost some of its legitimacy, it was in part because its practitioners erected a wall between themselves and the rest of society. But as internecine conflicts between specialties and organizations inside the field grew, physicians were less able to perceive their shared interests, and each organization also developed its own interests. Meanwhile, the decision-making power with regard to educational standards and licensure continued to reside with medical professionals.[155] Licensing boards made local decisions about exams, continuing medical education, and other requirements. In this climate, standardization and reciprocity could not be achieved.[156]

Criticism of licensing boards mounted in the 1960s, sometimes emanating from physicians. The AMA sounded its concern about the lack of board discipline,[157] and Dr. Derbyshire, a president of the Federation, took the lead in articulating the problem in medical journals and in his 1969 book, *Medical Licensure and Discipline in the United States*, which became known to the regulatory community for its insider critique.[158] He was among the first insiders to support limited public representation on medical boards. "Boards of medical examiners have not always operated properly and their conduct might well be subjected to more careful scrutiny. This could be accomplished by appointing a public member, who admittedly would possess no professional skills; for this reason he should not be allowed to vote on matters purely professional."[159] Derbyshire cited a board that had not revoked a license in twenty years, loopholes in medical acts that left opportunities for incompetents and imposters, and the citizenship requirement (in 1972 eight states required U.S. citizenship), which kept out qualified doctors. By 1974 he had answered his own question: "Are the boards of medical examiners adequately disciplining physicians, the answer must be, on the whole, no. The medical profession has long insisted that it can best police its own ranks, and it should. Yet unless all of the agencies involved in medical discipline work together to improve their methods, outsiders conceivably could take over the control of medical discipline. This must not happen."[160] He provided an insider's knowledge for public discussion of medical self-regulation.

The broader social, economic, and political environment was changing, too. State actors employed market rhetoric to spur consumer organizations. In 1962, President John F. Kennedy urged the empowerment of consumers: "Consumers, by definition, include us all. They are the largest economic group in the economy . . . and affected by almost every public and private economic decision. . . . But they are the only important groups in the economy who are not effectively organized, whose views are often not heard."[161]

By 1970, academic critics spurned appeals to professional altruism as self-serving and insincere; social scientists set out to show that professions were self-interested, concerned first and foremost with dominance and autonomy, market closure, imposition of their definition of needs and service on patients, and status maintenance.[162] Empirical studies of self-regulation multiplied, demonstrating that protection of the public interest cannot be left to professionals claiming to serve the public.[163] Freidson collected evidence that doctors did little informal regulation in their everyday practice.[164] Legislatures, supported by courts, had left the professions to their own devices, but this privilege was open to abuse. Insiders exposed the cracks in the professional community, but it took challenges by federal agencies to open a dialogue and start to develop new constituencies for boards—the state legislators, federal government, and general public.

Chapter 3

Public Participation

The Federal Bureaucracy Starts a Public Dialogue

George Bernard Shaw saw the medical profession as self interested: "[Medical practice] is quite unregulated except by professional etiquette, which, as we have seen, has for its object, not the health of the patient or of the community at large, but the protection of the doctor's livelihood and the concealment of his errors."[1] While Shaw's early criticism produced tangible results in 1926 in England with the addition of a public member to its medical regulatory board, the General Medical Council, in the United States, the issue of board accountability and public participation would not arise until the 1970s. It was not the public that forced the issue, but the federal government that opened the door to public dialogue and representation. Although the federal government encouraged civic involvement, it offered few incentives to facilitate state-level change.[2] But political currents of the 1960s and 1970s strengthened the resolve to change the system and brought an agenda of citizen participation forward.

This chapter focuses on discussions that laid out the rationale for public participation on state occupational regulatory boards.[3] The change in the regulatory climate reflected new trends in interest-group politics and participatory democracy of that era.[4] Debate on public participation came to a head in the 1970s at a time when reliance on experts and a professional self-governance philosophy came under attack from a coalition of progressive politicians, consumer-oriented activists, and academics calling on the federal agencies to enhance oversight.[5] The interest that the federal government took was economic—that is, to lower barriers to interstate mobility of labor and to reduce costs of medical care.[6] Public participation was one tool in the government's arsenal to compel doctors to open up the market.

Eliot Freidson considered the autonomy or ability to control one's working environment essential for professionals, yet the medical profession was not immune to the culture and political stirrings of the day. Civil rights, the drive toward local control of schools, consumer organizations' demands for the removal of unsafe cars—these signature movements of the 1960s created a climate in which it was harder for medical boards to continue to claim immunity from public scrutiny. In 1971, Dr. Robert McCleery's *One Life—One Physician: A Report to the Center for the Study of Responsive Law* spotlighted consumer safety issues plaguing the medical profession.[7]

The notion that experts know best what the public needs came under attack in the 1970s.[8] Leading the charge were women's health collectives, disability groups, complementary medicine practitioners, and self-help organizations.[9] Academics added their voices to the critical debate by exposing the medical profession's hunger for economic power and political influence.[10] With consumer groups clamoring for the independent evaluation of products and services, self-regulation and experts-know-best rhetoric fell on hard times.[11]

As radical consumer advocates called for administrative takeover and strong government regulation, many economists continued to press for deregulation, though neither took an extreme position for medicine.[12] State agencies increasingly acted as arbiters in disputes between competing interest groups. Voices previously excluded from the discussion found themselves welcome to debate. President Lyndon Johnson's Great Society programs reinforced the idea of public participation, which became the rallying cry for students demanding a share in university governance, community residents seeking local controls, citizens looking for representation on Model Cities boards, civilians securing membership on police review boards, and public representatives serving on health-planning agency boards.[13] Sensing the new political climate, the federal government stepped up its efforts to encourage public representation on state occupational regulatory boards.[14] In December 1976, with support from the Office of Consumer Affairs, the Federal Interagency Council on Citizen Participation held a two-day conference where two hundred staff members from about eighty government agencies referred to citizen engagement as a "fresh initiative."[15] James Creighton echoed the conference's main theme when he declared, "I believe citizen participation, public involvement—whatever you call it—is the adaptive response of our society to the demand for issue-by-issue accountability."[16]

Federal Government Agencies: Market Issues

When the U.S. Department of Labor got involved with licensure issues, it linked licensure to the need to facilitate interstate mobility of labor, which required eliminating unnecessary barriers of state licensing. The U.S. Department of Health, Education, and Welfare (HEW) also had its own agenda, including scope of practice issues, cost-effectiveness of different health-care providers, and federal government accountability for Medicare and Medicaid payments. The two federal departments came to see public membership as a boost to consumer confidence.[17] The U.S. Department of Education funded a newsletter of a citizens group dedicated to professional licensing issues—an important move given how little consumer discussions of licensing issues existed in the national arena. The challenge was to make occupations more responsive to market conditions by weakening the tight hold of professional associations on licensing boards.[18] The legitimacy of self-regulation emerged as an issue of discussion. No one questioned the notion that occupations should have a major say on how their fields were managed; the point was to make them accept the notion that their judgments were not above reproach.[19]

Title 1 of the Manpower Development and Training Act of 1962 directed the secretary of labor to investigate artificial barriers to labor market entry and mobility. In 1967 the Office of Research and Development of the Department of Labor gave a grant to Benjamin Shimberg to research barriers to interstate labor mobility and then to help states rewrite statutes to eliminate unnecessary requirements and to add public members to licensing boards.[20] Shimberg examined a range of licensing issues in various occupations but did not include doctors. However, he made numerous references to physicians, citing in particular a 1967 study by Forgotson, Roemer, and Newman, "Licensure of Physicians," which was a report of the National Advisory Commission on Health Manpower.[21] Medicine was one of many occupations under state jurisdiction that hampered interstate mobility.

According to Shimberg, public representation was one way to deal with problems of accountability. But public members lacked technical competence, could be outvoted, and had no constituency to look to for support. In contrast, a properly trained state representative could do a better job increasing accountability, Shimberg argued. In *Occupational Licensing: A Public Perspective* (1980), Shimberg evaluated public members' performance on occupational licensing boards in about thirty states. Board administrators said public members failed to attend after the first meetings because they felt excluded and intimidated by the technical skills of their professional counterparts, could not take time off from work, and were unsure about their role.[22] Still, Shimberg argued, public members could make a difference.[23] He also pushed hard for regulatory changes in state statutes. For thirteen years Shimberg persisted in his efforts, addressing state legislators, heads of regulatory agencies, governors' aides, attorneys general, and consumer advocates and providing technical information to reformers.[24] By 1980 Shimberg directly assisted thirty states and documented regulatory changes in thirty-six states, thus bringing public members into the political debate.[25]

The HEW mission included examining control over medical scope of practice issues to ensure that federal monies spent on Medicare and Medicaid would not be wasted on highly educated personnel when others could do the work. Harris S. Cohen of HEW authored several reports urging public participation as a means to increase medical boards' accountability, citing Shimberg and Robert Derbyshire.[26] The rationale for public participation, in his view, was not so much representing the public as a whole as adding a different voice to the review process.[27]

Although Congress commissioned the reports, it provided no financial incentives to states to encourage change. Cohen's HEW group did what a small dedicated group could be expected to do.[28] Independently, Cohen also criticized the licensing process, urging creation of boards with "a *substantial* number of public members."[29] In an article published in an academic journal he suggested that boards should be composed of members with no self-interest in the regulated profession, with physicians playing an advisory role.[30] The HEW report was particularly concerned about the conflict of interest endemic to self-regulation. "Submitting to 'community control' in the form of licensing has generally served to ensure the profession's freedom to control its own work. . . . The State licensing boards may work more or less discretely to present the profession's position regarding legislative proposals. In some States, professional associations work in conjunction with examining boards to initiate legislation, make additions or deletions, draft the preliminary and final proposed bills, persuade a legislator to introduce the bills, and then work for their passage."[31] The 1971 report issued by HEW strongly endorsed the idea of the "representation of consumers." More fodder for discussion was added in 1973 with a report titled "Developments in Health Manpower Licensure," which traced public-member participation to Governor Edmund "Pat" Brown, who had added community representatives to many California boards in 1961. But the report questioned the degree to which public members might increase the accountability of boards: "Of course, the very presence of lay members has probably tended to open up some of the secrecy attending board policy-making; but whether this is the sole function of public representation needs to be addressed, for the danger of token accountability lies in a facade of public reassurance, while permitting past practices to continue unabated."[32] Like Shimberg, some feared public participation would remain largely ceremonial.

A third draft report was made public in 1976, and drew a heated response from the medical profession. In its early version, the report grouped medicine with the allied health professions, but the final 1977 report discarded this categorization and recommended national certification for allied health professions—not medicine.[33] The 1976 draft did not mention public participation, but the final report did.

In 1977 the Department of Education (Office of Consumer Education) provided funding to the National Center for the Study of Professions whose primary goal was to develop a network of people involved with professional regulatory boards. The center published a newsletter, *ProForum*, that helped cement an alliance among organizations working to improve professional regulation.[34] It also provided an additional outlet, *The Public Member*, that reached out to public members throughout the 1980s. Its publications ensured that professional regulation would remain a topic for discussion.

The federal government reports raised doubts about the claims that boards worked to protect the public interest in the economic arena. Labor has to be reasonably free to move where the opportunities beckoned; federal dollars should not be wasted on overqualified personnel; and the public ought to have a say on economic and safety issues. Although the AMA challenged boards to improve efficiency, it did not challenge board legitimacy. Federal agencies, however, could do little more than try to persuade state groups to take action. Little was said at first about physician misconduct.

Competing Interests of Medical Organizations

Fears of federal involvement for both the AMA and FSMB were critical, but the FSMB began slowly to accept public members as boards saw their legitimacy at stake. The AMA spoke strongly against public participation at first but then removed many doctors from board purview by creating diversionary programs for doctors with substance abuse and mental health issues. The bulk of the profession remained unenthusiastic about the prospect of having nonexperts challenging their judgment but did not believe public members would have much impact.

Doctors tended to see themselves as professionals distinguished by their expertise, good character, and impartiality, which, taken together, separated them from other occupations. We can see this sentiment in a 1925 AMA report that enshrined medical expertise as essential for both technical and moral decisions: "Statutes prescribing the requisite regulation of the doctor's occupation will not enforce themselves. Neither are they enforceable by the ordinary public officers charged with general administration of the laws. . . .

They must conduct examinations in scientific subjects and scientific technic that can be conducted only by experts in those matters. . . . They must possess and apply accurate judgment of the moral qualifications of applicants in admitting persons to the doctor's occupation."[35] Lack of medical knowledge on the part of the public led the AMA to decry the idea of public participation and throw their support behind "peer review."

Physicians understood that their interests were better protected by state rather than federal regulation. For example, some members of the FSMB in 1916, during a discussion of the National Board of Medical Examiners and national standards, expressed fear of the federal government: "Dr. T. J. Crowe of Dallas also took a dim view of the National Board [NBME], darkly hinting that it was a step towards federal control of licensure; this, despite the repeated protestation of the founders of the National Board that it only sought to be a voluntary qualifying body."[36] That fear of national licensure remained in 1976 and made the Federation and AMA unhappy with the HEW draft report recommendations—subsuming physicians under the category of "health professionals," with calls for national certification that seemed more threatening than public participation.[37] The draft was greeted with several hundred letters expressing concern about national licensure.[38] Medical organizations worked to negotiate changes in the final HEW report.

The final 1977 report changed "health occupations" to "allied health occupations"—a designation aimed to decouple physicians from other health professionals. Wherever "federal government" was mentioned in the draft, "state government" was put in its place. To relieve the apprehension of many physicians that national credentialing meant federal licensing, the final report stated: "It is important to emphasize that the development and adoption of national standards should not be confused with Federal licensure. Licensure is presently, and will continue to be, a function of State government."[39] The report readded the importance of consumers, which was not in the draft.[40] But fears of federal involvement remained. Jackson Riddle, MD, PhD, and director of AMA Division of Educational Policy and Development, wrote in 1976, "The threat of federal licensure . . . evoked an unfavorable reaction little short of unanimous."[41] The AMA showed its fear of federal involvement in a lawsuit it filed against professional standards review organization (PSRO) regulations.[42] Medical organizations preferred public participation to federal involvement.[43]

Despite AMA objections, FSMB slowly accepted the limited presence of public members as a way to shore up its public standing. Dr. Stein, board member from California, praised public members in 1968: "The 11 professional members . . . working for the best interests of the public and the medical profession. . . . The one lay member of the board has also consistently advocated policies which will uphold the standards of medical excellence and he has been most helpful in discussions of matters pertaining to the functions of the board."[44]

But the AMA remained tentative about public members. Dr. Charles Hoffman, president of the AMA, addressed a Federation gathering in 1973: "We recommend that licensing boards have public representation on the boards. Now I know California does have one public representative. He is an attorney. . . . My experience with the Blue Shield boards is that the consumer members, the public members, are a great help as long as they are *informed* public members. . . . So I see nothing wrong with having possibly one consumer, one public member, on licensing boards."[45] The AMA did not fully support that view. In 1978 Dr. John Budd, AMA president, opposed public participation in the following terms: "Only professionals can police their ranks competently and knowledgeably. . . . I think our profession is also being undermined by vehement forms of consumerism."[46]

In 1969 Dr. Derbyshire of FSMB had argued that public members would legitimate board decisions without making much impact: "To many members of medical boards as well as to the medical association, my advocacy of the inclusion of a non medical member on boards is nothing short of heresy. My point is that the primary function of the boards is to protect the public. They are public bodies and should have public representation. . . . I am unable to understand, however, how more than one or two public members could contribute much to a board with such highly technical functions."[47] The next year, however, he sounded alarmed about the prospect of public members gaining too strong a footing on medical boards: "The medical profession has long insisted that it can best police its own ranks, and it should. . . . Outsiders conceivably could take over control of medical discipline. This must not happen."[48]

The Federation was not especially worried about public legitimacy, for it saw physicians as its only constituency. In his 1970 editorial, Dr. F. Merchant, president of the FSMB, wrote: "Medical licensing boards in general need to negate an unfortunate stigma which has become attached to many of them, namely, that of being gray-haired uncomprehending reactionaries bent on obstructing rather than meeting change. The sooner board members grasp the significance of this stigma, the better will be their relationships with medical schools, medical associations, and other medical boards."[49]

It was only a matter of time before the FSMB saw the wisdom of incorporating more of the protect-the-public rhetoric into its discourse. The next

Federation president, Frank Edmondson, MD, wrote: "While it is true that the primary role of the state boards is to determine the qualifications of those about to enter professional practice, it is equally true that the boards have the obligation to protect the public from those who have become incompetent to practice because of age, illness, or professional obsolescence."[50] In 1975 Dr. John Morton, member of FSMB journal editorial board, claimed: "There is a growing feeling that there should be public members on state licensing boards. Advocates of this position believe that boards, as presently constituted, act to protect the profession rather than the public. . . . They feel that, if the public is ably and vocally represented, the boards will deal more responsibly with their charge. . . . What is the disadvantage inherent in having public representation on the board?"[51] By the mid-1970s "protecting the public" became a staple issue for the medical boards articulating their mission statements. At last, the boards began to include the public as their intended audience, even if only a passive one.

Legitimacy became more important. During his 1975 FSMB presidential address Dr. Howard Horns had this to say: "Recent legislation provided for three public members. . . . Our appraisal led us to expect that public members might provide a communication channel and prevent a great deal of misunderstanding and suspicion. We believe that professional members may be made more accurately aware of public attitudes and expectations and that statements of the board may be presented without suspicion of self interest."[52]

Public members gained voice in the FSMB. In 1977 Sherwin J. Memel, JD, became president of the California board,[53] and a California physician board member wrote: "State boards should have the benefit of intelligent minority participation. At the last annual meeting [FSMB] there were several representatives of the public, particularly one newspaper editor, who voiced his opinion and encouraged the Federation to suggest that all states attempt to comply with this idea that minority and public representation should be present on state boards."[54] Some FSMB physicians saw public members as contributing to decisions: "They have participated actively in board affairs. (2) Since they bring a different point of view to board discussion, their insights have strengthened board decisions. (3) They have dispelled the myth that the board acts only to protect the physician, neglecting its duty to the public. (4) They have demonstrated that medical board activities are responsibly conducted and can withstand public scrutiny."[55] An important change in the Federation by-laws came in 1982 when a director at large—a nonphysician—was added to its board.[56]

Looking back at the tortuous process that led the medical profession to endorse the idea of public representation, we can see that physicians were in large measure responsible for opening themselves to regulatory strictures. By showing the reluctance to discuss the boards' problems openly,[57] the FSMB raised concerns about the willingness and ability of physicians to discipline their own.[58] By the time the boards realized they needed public members to fend off further regulatory oversight, they invited scrutiny from state agencies. Even then, public members felt unwelcome on many boards. California, however, cancelled its FSMB membership for a short period to encourage the FSMB to include public members on its board.[59] The medical profession stood to lose self-regulation altogether, and this is one reason why the profession accepted public participation, albeit reluctantly.[60] And public members would be largely ceremonial, a point with which many academics who studied professions would concur, as the profession controlled the discourse.[61]

The AMA still claimed that its expertise required self-regulation. Specialized knowledge implied peer review, for no one else could understand what it takes to practice medicine. The judicial council of the AMA explained, "At every plane, discipline is administered by physicians in discharge of their professional responsibility to society. This is peer review in the finest sense."[62] In 1980, AMA President Dr. Hoyt Gardner invoked the "peer review" option in his FSMB address: "Professional regulation will remain in the hands of people like us. . . . The AMA has long been a champion of conscientious peer review . . . the medical profession should safeguard the public and itself against physicians deficient in moral character or professional competence."[63]

If the knowledge was so complex and identification, diagnosis, and treatment a learned "art," it would be difficult for an outsider to assess the quality of the diagnosis or treatment.[64] The extent to which expertise was truly an insurmountable issue remained unclear. However, many problems facing the boards revolved around ethical concerns and access issues—squarely within the public domain. Insistence on expertise served as an obstacle to democratic processes by disempowering nonexperts.[65] The medical profession had used its power to corner the market, jack up its status, and control peoples' bodies and lives.[66]

New Organizations: Impaired Physicians Programs

In examining disciplinary statistics available in the 1960s, physicians realized most of those disciplined could be removed from board scrutiny and managed within the medical community. Between 1963 and 1967, of 938 licensure actions nationally, 646 were for narcotics use, mental incompetence, abortions, and alcoholism.[67] The medical profession met the challenge with the development of independent "self-reporting" tracks for "impaired physicians."[68] In the

1970s and 1980s medical societies, sometimes with boards, established organizations to direct the rehabilitation of chemically dependent (drugs and alcohol) and mentally disabled physicians, with some states adding sexual offenders.[69] Since the 1960s, many doctors and the public considered chemical dependency a medical issue that legitimated physician-supervised treatment.[70]

The AMA board of trustees approved "The Disabled Physician Act" in 1974, arguing that impaired physicians needed effective rehabilitation, not punishment. The AMA act was designed to place the "medical society in the role of the agent for the licensing body in examining the physician in question and making recommendation on treatment and remedial action [and to] ensure effective treatment and rehabilitation."[71] The state medical societies responded, often with board support, by establishing impaired physicians programs (IPPs), supervised by impaired physician committees (IPCs) to protect and rehabilitate physicians, thus potentially diverting physicians from the disciplinary process and board purview.

Claiming that confidentiality was necessary to encourage self-reporting, the medical establishment successfully fought to establish complete confidentiality for those "voluntarily" enrolled in programs. The licenses of doctors enrolled remained unencumbered in many states, and treatment providers decided whether physicians should practice while undergoing treatment and when they could return to practice. Confidentiality for voluntary admissions was assured in California: "The names of participants who have been ordered into the Diversion Program as part of a disciplinary action are public record. The statutes establishing the Diversion Program require confidentiality of all other participants who enter the program voluntarily."[72] Another board appeared to go further with the goal of confidentiality. A 1997 Nevada medical board newsletter stated: "Self referrals are extremely rare. . . . Most come from partners or colleagues, hospitals or through law enforcement channels. . . . Physicians are also referred to diversion when undergoing board investigation for other matters and an impairment is suspected. In all cases, no records are kept at board level. . . . [This] will further separate the diversion program operation from other board activities and protect anonymity of participants."[73]

Even in states with a cooperative agreement with the medical boards, most of the authority rested with the impairment programs to supervise and make decisions. In Florida, the medical society and the board each tried to set up programs and joined in 1985 to set up a recovery network. In 1995 an IPP staff member wrote: "Prior to the collaboration, the regulatory agency's program was misperceived as too public and punitive, and the medical association's program was perceived as secretive and an extension of the 'conspiracy of silence.'"[74] About 84 percent of the people in the program entered before they violated the medical practice act. Although the program could suspend a license temporarily if the doctor posed an immediate threat to the public, the decision rested with the program, not the board. Either informally or formally, the programs made most of the decisions concerning doctors enrolled.

The relatively weak ties between the boards and the programs raise concerns. In 1989 the Oregon legislature created a diversion program where participants signed voluntary agreements and were monitored in recovery.[75] Nevertheless, "The goal is to confidentially offer access to diagnostic, treatment and recovery programs, without board intervention or board knowledge" in order to encourage early entry into treatment.[76] The director of the program explained that of the forty-eight licensees treated between 1990 and 1993, only two were turned over to the disciplinary board and relapsed into "persistent" chemical use. But: "If someone does experience relapse, we don't look at that as failure. Part of the disease of substance abuse can be relapse. . . . The last thing we want to do is turn a relapsed licensee over to the board for disciplinary action because then no one wins."[77] Except, perhaps, the patients.

Stronger supervisory relationships by some boards of the impaired physician programs did not deter self-referrals. Missouri sent anonymous reports on all physicians in its impairment program to the board when the board and the medical society started working together in 1985. If a doctor sent by the board relapsed, the program became his advocate in front of the board.[78] A few states mandated protection of the public as the primary goal. Washington State passed a bill in 1988 in which the legislature stipulated that protection of the public was the program's primary responsibility.[79] At least symbolically, some programs acknowledged the importance of public protection.

To develop program standards, the Federation appointed a committee in 1993, and the report, accepted by the Federation in 1995, documented how a program should be set up but did not take a stand on whether the board should be informed about a self-reporting physician or what the relationship between the IPC and the board should be. The committee did not address the tensions between possible disparate goals.[80] The argument that strict confidentiality is key to self-referral and rehabilitation rationalizes a weak link between the boards and the programs. If we look at the statistics furnished by the programs—90 percent of the physicians enrolled in the programs are reported as rehabilitated—we may think that the public may appear reasonably protected.[81] But the secrecy in which most programs operate means that the public must trust the programs to ensure that doctors do not practice "in the name of treatment" when impaired. Program goals are treatment and rehabilitation, not public protection.

The tension between "rehabilitation" and "protecting the public" was addressed at a conference convened by the public interest group Citizen Advocacy Center (CAC) in March 1998. The split between the rehabilitative community and board members was significant. Board members angered treatment representatives when they said that IPPs and licensing boards had different interests. After a presenter made an argument for patients' rights and safety, an IPP staff member averred that he "would definitely choose the person in recovery as my surgeon." Clapping erupted. Impassioned applause broke out again when a treatment provider started his comment with "I go back thirty years when there was nothing and lots of bad ideas." Dead silence met a board member's comment that it was necessary to discuss possible conflicts between the confidentiality (from the boards) the recovery programs demanded and public protection. When a board member said that permitting a doctor to continue to practice when he had "dirty urine" might put the public at risk, a treatment provider responded, "I can make an assessment about when the board needs to know." Some treatment program staff never acknowledged even the possibility of a conflict. As chair of the Florida medical society's judicial council put it in 1975, rehabilitation's primary goal is "the protection of the dignity and honor of the profession."[82] Recovery programs sometimes conflate protecting the public with getting the physician back into practice through a treatment regimen. Loyalty is to their "patients"—doctors in recovery—and not the public who may be treated by someone during a relapse. Treatment programs do an important job of rehabilitating impaired physicians, but public protection is the work of medical boards, and they need to be involved.

Public advocates, some board members, and some board staff sounded an alarm about this state of affairs and advocated an alternative at the CAC conference. One public advocate asked, "What happens to patients' rights?" A board staff member pointed out that some physician drug users also sell or steal drugs. A board member described a doctor who took pain medication from patients and used it himself. If board members are to put patient safety first, they must be more involved in the decision about when a doctor should practice during recovery.

In some states sexual misconduct cases are handled by IPPs. For instance, the North Carolina medical society and the board wrote a statute in 1987 that permitted the board to form an IPP and designated the medical society to run the program.[83] Of the first 500 cases, 38 involved sexual misconduct and 338 involved chemical dependency. In some states, sexual misconduct can be self-reported to the program; in others, the board sends sexual offenders for rehabilitation after the board takes action. A Federation committee took a strong stand in 1995 that most sexual offenders should be disciplined and could not be rehabilitated, as sexual misconduct was not a mental illness.[84] While the medical profession diverted many impaired physicians and successfully rehabilitated a significant group, thus maintaining patient access, with secrecy from boards, they potentially made decisions placing rehabilitation over patient safety.

State Medical Societies Object to Public Members

More than autonomy and self-governance were at issue in the medical profession's opposition to outside review. The world of medicine was rife with conflicts of interest that undermined the profession's ability to police itself through self-regulation. The articles in medical publications supporting professional control over board issues continued to appear in the 1970s and 1980s. The key argument in defense of self-regulation was the lack of expertise of public members.

In several states the medical societies took a more forceful stance against public members than the AMA. The perceived threat of national licensure had been settled as far as the AMA was concerned, and local medical societies were left to concentrate on managing the increasing interest of the media and state bureaucracies in licensing. The mounting pressure on medical professionals can be gleaned from an editorial published in a medical journal whose author lamented that the regulatory innovations were "most often stimulated by pressures arising outside the profession. These pressures may emanate from a dissatisfied segment of the public, or the public press. . . . All too rarely are the laws rewritten at the request of the profession."[85] In 1972 the *Illinois Medical Journal* harped on public representatives who were asked to render judgments for which they lacked qualifications: "It has been proposed that the state add public representation on all health profession examining committees to reflect the needs of consumers and other health care providers and ensure greater public accountability for committee actions. Advocates of this proposal contend that the addition of well-qualified laymen . . . would provide checks and balances and lessen the possibility of arbitrary committee decisions. . . . ISMS [the Illinois State Medical Society] questions the advisability of public members on examining committees."[86] This staunch opposition achieved its goal—when two consumers were appointed to the disciplinary board, they were denied the right to vote. This ban continued until 1987, the year when the legislature raised the number of public members on the disciplinary board to four. Both boards were reconstituted as largely advisory to a state agency.

"Peer review" was the mantra of medical societies; bureaucratic meddling was anathema. The president of the Medical Association of Georgia (MAG), Dr. C. E. Bohler, maintained that board actions amounted to "peer review," with the board acting as an extension of the medical society: "All agree that physicians can best scrutinize other physicians. The Attorney General negated our plans. There is no provision in the Medical Practice Act for such actions by the State Board. . . . We will not give up . . . provide peer investigation. . . . The idea of peer investigation will, in many instances, cause a wayward physician to straighten up and fly right. . . . MAG is enjoying excellent rapport with and the full cooperation of the board."[87] It was difficult to pass public interest legislation when the medical society and boards were so closely aligned. In 1976 Dr. W. J. Morton was executive director of the medical board and member of MAG committee on legislation, and no public members were added when the Medical Practice Act was passed with the enthusiastic support of the MAG. Others emphasized the importance of bringing "justice to a wrong doer . . . knowing that the effort will in fact preserve and protect our right and responsibility to police and protect our honored profession."[88] Despite these antiregulatory sentiments, Georgia did admit one public member in 1979, but unlike many other states, added no additional members. Public accountability was not a major issue for the society's members.

Even after North Carolina added public members, the board appeared to remain firmly under medical control. The medical society chose the board members, and, as late as 1988, the board chair, Dr. E. Alexander, did not acknowledge the public member appointed seven years earlier. "The members of the board feel they represent all of medicine, and in point of fact are dealing with standard of care and the management of patients."[89] They later added more public members. So far as many medical societies were concerned, boards' sole constituency was the medical community despite the discourse of national organizations that began to acknowledge the public as a constituency.

The transition of boards to focus on discipline, include public members, work more within state bureaucracies, and increase transparency was not an easy process and varied significantly from state to state. Some boards have made very few changes, and others have evolved considerably into the twenty-first century. But a central question for the profession remains to be answered: Does public members' participation remain chiefly ceremonial, or is it capable of making a difference in the decision-making process?

Chapter 4

The State, the Media, and the Shaping of Public Opinion

Local medical societies often resisted changes, yielding only when media campaigns grew too hot and when boards found they had less to do since licensure issues were largely resolved by the use of national exams.[1] As George Bernard Shaw argued in the 1930s, "In the main, then, the doctor learns that if he gets ahead of the superstitions of his patients he is a ruined man; and the result is that he instinctively takes care not to get ahead of them. That is why all the changes came from the laity."[2] The 1980s saw a gradual decoupling of boards from medical societies. Whatever the regulatory agenda national authorities had in mind, they had to coordinate with local associations, the media, the public, and state legislatures and agencies.

Constituencies often emerge in response to specific issues brought to their attention by the media, which plays a vital role in mobilizing public attention in defense of its interests. Some credit for making the public aware of its stake in the regulation game belongs to scholars like Benjamin Shimberg, who worked with local consumer groups and sensitized state government agencies about the deficiencies in the regulatory process. Media exposés and editorials were consistent with these critiques. Dr. Sidney Wolfe, director of the Public Citizen Health Research Group, wrote in 1993 that "despite the seriousness of many of these offenses, the licenses of the physicians who committed them are often neither revoked nor suspended and many of these doctors are practicing medicine, seeing patients who are completely in the dark about what the state boards have concluded. . . . The patients who go to these doctors have a right to know more about them than they can read in the yellow pages."[3]

Once discipline became the focus and the media took it upon itself to "define an issue and to create a story,"[4] local publics grew increasingly alarmed about the lack of disciplinary action against errant doctors. Legislators, especially those in states with sunset legislation, which mandated review of agencies, could not ignore the negative board coverage in the media, whose harangues shaped as well as served to express public opinion. Adding public members to medical boards seemed like the least legislators could do to mollify public opinion. With public members the question arose as to their qualifications and proper role. Public-interest groups took up this question and supported government agencies in their agenda to push boards to pursue quality-of-care (negligence and incompetence) cases more aggressively. As the number of disciplinary actions grew, the courts increasingly found themselves drawn into the fray, particularly by due-process issues.[5] Responding to public outrage, legislators began to weigh in on the lack of oversight, and some demanded not only public members on boards and increased transparency but incorporating boards more into state bureaucracies.

By the twenty-first century, the public in many states had evolved into a constituency that had to be reckoned with. Activists and citizen groups demanded to know why doctors continued to practice in one state after they lost licenses in others, how many malpractice suits it took for a doctor to be deemed unfit, and what the reasons were behind the wide range of disciplinary actions taken among in different jurisdictions. To understand how these questions were raised and answered, we need to examine how public opinion was mobilized with the help of the media in defense of patients' interests.

The division of labor between state and public actors in the early public dialogue advocating for change was fuzzy. With funding from the U.S. Department of Labor, Shimberg worked for Educational Testing Service and tried to sell the idea of public board members directly to states. *ProForum*, a newsletter dedicated to improving professional regulation, was written by a public-interest group (the National Center for the Study of Professions) funded by the U.S. Department of Education. Common Cause, another public-interest group, pushed sunset legislation as a response to the possible overexpansion of government regulation and thereby could provide an opportunity for change.[6] The 1976 Colorado sunset legislation mandated regular state review of agencies and demonstration of accountability. Most of the thirty-six states that passed sunset legislation did so between 1976 and 1980. National consumer groups kept licensing boards under close scrutiny. In 1978, a conference on licensing sponsored by COCO (the Conference of Consumer Organizations, formed in 1973) included nonprofit consumer groups and government agencies that promoted public members.[7]

Sunset legislation provided an opportunity to promote public scrutiny and legislative oversight. Shimberg suggested issues for the public to raise about boards for sunset reviews. Among them were "Are boards fully autonomous or have efforts been made to place restrictions on their power? . . . Do boards seem to be serving the public or occupational group? . . . Urge the legislature to make adequate resources available to support enforcement activities. . . . Seek legislation that will make it easier to identify 'high risk' practitioners. . . . Insist that publicity be given to disciplinary action against licensees. . . . Has the board sought to involve the public in its meetings?"[8]

To their credit, state agencies and legislators acknowledged that public-interest groups expressed public perspectives. The *ProForum* newsletter reaffirmed the importance of sunset to licensing reform: "Common Cause recommends that regulatory agencies be the first target of Sunset reviews because of their heavy impact on the economy and because 'they are a source of much citizen dissatisfaction with government.'"[9] *ProForum* quoted David Cohen, president of Common Cause, who favored open-meeting requirements and independent-minded public members.[10] In that same 1980 issue *ProForum* also quoted President Jimmy Carter addressing a White House conference on regulatory reform: "Many regulatory agencies at the state and local levels . . . protect monopolies."[11] According to a 1986 survey response from twenty-eight states, sunset legislation had a tangible effect as evidenced by the addition of public members (eighteen states), increased disciplinary and investigative functions (sixteen states), and improved complaint handling (seventeen states). In many cases, these changes were opposed by medical societies.[12]

An Active Media

Medical boards' failures to discipline doctors make great local headlines.[13] Several such investigative series reflected the reporting tradition of Watergate. "So long as information is publicly available," observed Michael Schudson, "political actors have to behave *as if* someone in the public is paying attention."[14] Investigative reporting not only spotlighted hidden problems but also helped clarify the issues and identify key players responsible for the problems and their solutions. The media glare neutralized the clout of medical societies and their ability to obfuscate the issues and put pressure on legislatures to take action. By expounding on the "duty" of legislators and governors and citing their statements in support of reform, the press increased the accountability of public officials. Some investigations led to changes in the practice acts that were a direct result of the reporters' allegations.[15] Media attention did not always mobilize the public, but some constituents pressured legislators to take action.[16]

Sunset procedures also facilitated change by requiring board evaluations by legislative committees, and, in the wake of media exposés, legislatures were pushed to make more drastic changes. Reporters provided citizens with their first critical views into medical organizations and laid groundwork for future public activism. In this climate, citizens were more likely to exchange views on relevant issues, call a legislator, report an errant physician, or start a public-interest group. The media emerged as a key player in promoting the need for new regulatory tools and oversight of the medical profession.[17] A story might focus on a particular event, but it also made the public aware of the wide range of players in the regulation game.[18]

A Pulitzer Finalist and Sunset: Radical Change in Florida

The power of sunset provisions is evident in the case of the Florida board, which lost its autonomy to a centralized agency and was compelled to add public members after the public read a 1980 Pulitzer finalist investigation in the *Miami Herald* in 1979 that led to the Department of Professional Regulation takeover of disciplinary investigations and prosecutions.[19] A legislative insider described to *ProForum* the position of the board: "The articles created a volatile and negative atmosphere. Rather than meeting the criticism head-on, the board members tried stone-walling on the basis of their meritorious position as doctors, said Gary Van Ostrand, former staff director of the house subcommittee on regulatory reform which oversees Sunset review. . . . 'Quite frankly, the board was caught with its pants down.'"[20] The sunset committee held public hearings for the board to answer the charges, after which the board requested additional rules to facilitate prosecution and a toll-free complaint number.

The series included a dazzling array of articles describing mangled patients, unfit doctors, sex with patients, alcohol abuse, drug addiction, and pedophilia—plenty to fan the public's worst fears. The eight-day series included headlines such as "Why Bad Doctors Get Away with It,"[21] "Patient: He Forced Me to Have Sex,"[22] and "Discipline by Board Is Lenient."[23] Many complaints about dangerous doctors came from other doctors. The series also revealed the board's limited ability to manage cases owing to lack of resources, fear of lawsuits, and the informal code of silence among doctors. An editorial urged the dismissal of the executive director, the release of board members from their duties, the addition of public members to the board, an increase in licensure fees, the creation of a "sick doctor" program, publication of future board actions, and requiring insurance companies to notify boards by about malpractice settlements.[24] This media exposure put pressure on the legislature to reform board procedures. Two months later, the paper quoted a legislator: "Dunn said that a recent *Miami Herald* series of stories revealing chronic disciplinary problems in the medical profession 'got the ball rolling' toward a legislative overhaul of professional discipline."[25] And seven months later an article stated, "Shocked law makers gutted the old Florida board . . . removing nearly all of its staff and much of its power."[26] The organization was pulled within the state bureaucracy.

Despite changes, the physicians continued to talk mainly to each other. Even before the 1979 news series, the board and the medical society sought to explain the problems to their medical constituents. Dr. Vernon Astler, board president, in 1974 wrote an "open letter to Representative Forbes" in response to a *Jacksonville Journal* article criticizing the board. The president insisted, "The board of Medical Examiners does not act as a 'buffer' to 'keep out people' . . . we are a consumer protection agency and to this end our role is to determine that only properly qualified and competent MD's are allowed the privilege of licensure."[27] The next year, Dr. G. S. Palmer, executive director of the board, defended the board while referring to a critical news article "and increased involvement—and meddling—of idealistic planners and do-gooders in medical affairs. . . . Each of us also is a custodian of the House of Medicine, and we are responsible for keeping it in order. If we don't rise to this challenge, who will?"[28] W. W. Thompson, MD, chair of the medical association judicial council, emphasized the rehabilitative possibilities of the board to the profession: "The protection of the public from the menace or threat of an unqualified or mentally or physically disabled practitioner is a prime consideration. But if there is a chance that the man might be shown the error of his ways and restored to useful service some day, that must be taken into account. . . . There is a third consideration, and that is the protection of the dignity and honor of the profession. Bringing the errant practitioner to terms and making him mend his way if it is possible to do so removes a blight on all of us."[29] After the passage of new legislation, the medical society sought to put a positive spin on the changes.[30] As usual, the profession addressed its immediate constituency—the physicians. The optimistic messages notwithstanding, a second series of articles appeared in 1982 in the *St. Petersburg Times*, providing details of drug abuse, botched surgeries, sex exploitation, and drug trafficking. The board and the regulatory agency were blamed for their failure to follow up on cases and clean up the mess. The situation got worse, according to the story, because the doctors' registration fees had been cut, leaving the board with fewer resources for investigation and discipline.[31]

Dr. R. J. Feinstein, appointed board director after the passage of the new statute, explained the legislative changes to his colleagues brought about after the 1979 *Miami Herald* series. The board was reorganized to include nine doctors and two public members. He pointed out a 1981 *Wall Street Journal* article that singled out the Florida board as particularly effective.[32] Public members served as a source of legitimacy, but two years later, Dr. Feinstein offered an additional function: "Public members should continue to serve on boards to offer a nonphysician's perspective on the disciplinary process and to allay public anxiety. . . . The profession seeks to maintain its integrity and independence from bureaucratic control, and the state seeks to protect its citizens from incompetent practitioners and from monopolistic behavior, such as exclusion of new practitioners and the control of fees."[33] With the conflict of interests in full view, some within the profession began to address the public directly, recognizing it as a legitimate constituency.[34]

Sunset and the Medical Society Went Down Fighting: Texas

In Texas, the press played a role in thwarting the board's effort to shield itself from negative publicity. The Texas Medical Association (TMA) had a history of opposing practice act changes. The state passed sunset legislation in 1977 but did not evaluate the medical practice act until 1982. According to *ProForum*, the Texas board would cease operation on September 12, 1982, as legislators failed to agree on reauthorization. In intense political maneuvering, the Sunset Commission recommended adding public members to the board, stronger conflict-of-interest provisions, tighter state budget controls, and other good government measures. Yet the bill was introduced neither in the senate nor the house. The controversy that swept the senate concerned public members and osteopathic physicians. "The public member issue was settled after the TMA agreed not to oppose any bill which called for public representation."[35]

The legislative fight was widely reported in Texas, according to *ProForum:* "The *Houston Chronicle* reported that TMA's chief lobbyist said that the association would 'destroy' any legislator who opposed the association's position." Robert Morris, a member of the Sunset Commission staff, told *ProForum*: "They [the TMA] antagonized everyone with their self-importance and arrogance. The legislature is like a club with a select membership, and it became embarrassing to support TMA. . . . The doctors just do not understand how these things work. . . . The speaker appointed himself to the conference committee because he was upset by TMA's attitude."[36] The TMA efforts to block legislation backfired.[37]

Shortly before the legislature opened the practice act under sunset provisions again in 1993, not only did a 1992 media exposé by Ruth Sorelle in the *Houston Chronicle* criticize both the TMA and the board, but it also stated that legislators and the governor were concerned about board failures, making it difficult for them not to push for changes. The legislation added three public members to increase their board percentage from 20 percent to 33 percent. Not only the press, but also a physician and two public members took pains to publicize the board's failures. They were quoted as saying that the public interest received short shrift. The exposé also reported incidents of failure to revoke Texas licenses when other states had done so, failure to sanction doctors found guilty of felony offenses, and failure to revoke licenses of doctors who violated probation conditions. "'We are not a disciplinary board,' said Pharo [president of the board], who resigned shortly after being interviewed. 'We are actually a regulatory board.'"[38] The article explained that most decisions were made in informal settlement conferences without prosecution or a public member present. It also quoted a member of Public Citizen on cases of felony convictions: "It's not in the board's purview to go second guessing a criminal court. That's obviously horrendous." The legislators took note of the article, and the chair of the Sunset Commission was quoted as saying, "That's the trouble with the good ol' boy deal. They don't think a doctor could do that."

The investigative reporter reviewed 216 cases dismissed at informal settlement conferences over three years and reported that; "the board's representatives repeatedly disregarded complaints against doctors who had already been determined to have rendered substandard care by the Texas Medical Foundation, a review group that evaluated treatment of Medicare patients; doctors who have been removed from the staffs of hospitals because of poor patient care; or doctors who had been found to prescribe excessive quantities of drugs."[39] The board staff was also found wanting—one told a board in another state that a doctor's license was unencumbered several years after he had been sanctioned. The board attorney explained the decision to exclude a parent of a dead child from the hearing as this might inject "an emotional element that would perhaps be undesirable."[40]

Board members' statements further exposed the board's ineffectiveness and uncritical commitment to a rehabilitation philosophy that kept the board from revoking licenses. According to one story, a physician board member observed, "We have 340 doctors on probation. How can anybody expect us to have two people monitoring that many and making sure that everything is kosher?" A public member then said, "We don't have any teeth in our probation," and another one stated, "Some doctors [on the board] seem to think that their job is to reform these doctors. But we don't have enough staff. . . . If we can rehabilitate that physician, it's just lagniappe." When asked why he was unconcerned about a physician continuing his work while on probation for substance abuse, the board president said, "He's not a bad doctor. He's a bad person."[41]

Another news article discussed specific changes. Both public members on this board supported an increase in public membership to one-third, and another member wanted to depoliticize the process of choosing members. Despite documentation of serious problems, the board president claimed that the current process was fine. The lawyer who drafted the practice act in 1982 served as defense lawyer for physicians before the board: "He is so successful that board members have secretly referred doctors [under investigation by the board] to him themselves."[42] No one appeared to be watching out for the public.

A month later, the Sunset Commission was about to release its report when the newspaper spread the news that the governor sought greater public representation on the board and urged an overhaul of the entire monitoring system. The paper reminded the public, the legislature, and the governor that something had to be done;[43] it engaged in public dialogue with the profession, the state, and the public members, goading the legislators into action. By discussing board problems and reminding legislators that they promised reform, the paper, representing a public constituency, directly held the legislators accountable.

The Massachusetts Medical Society Steps Up

In 1992 many articles appeared in the *Boston Globe* on the medical board and its relationship to the Dr. Margaret Bean-Bayog case, a psychiatrist whose patient, a medical student, committed suicide in April 1991. The paper alleged an improper doctor-patient relationship and that the psychiatrist wrote to the patient about her fantasies. Besides captivating the public, the story put the spotlight on the work of a grossly underfunded and understaffed board that failed to manage its cases properly. The board director was fired. When Bean-Bayog surrendered her license, the case had not yet been heard by the board, as the reporter in the *Boston Globe* pointed out on September 18, 1992.[44]

Problems for the board were not over. The *Boston Globe* reported on March 11, 1993, that a public member was elected chair, and the Massachusetts Medical Society "regretted the appointment but would continue to 'work cooperatively' with the board." According to a board physician, "To protect the consumer, we have to have the ability to reach doctors and get them to cooperate with us. . . . By having a non-physician chair, we may lose that ability and this move may be counterproductive." Another doctor claimed that lawyers would never allow a nonlawyer on their disciplinary committee.[45]

During October 1994, the *Boston Globe* published a series of articles claiming that hospitals were not reporting losses of hospital privileges and major adverse outcomes to the medical board as required by law. Additionally, a public advocacy group criticized the board for tabling a proposal to make malpractice information publicly available.[46] Two articles described the board as backing off the reform and the medical society being as "antipublic" in its insistence that malpractice history was not something the patient should be concerned about.[47] The articles about medical board issues continued to appear regularly in the *Boston Globe*, fanning the complaints about too few disciplinary actions,[48] the lack of public information on problem doctors,[49] and the alarming rates of hospital mistakes.[50]

The board's activities were brought directly to the attention of the Massachusetts legislature when the state Teachers Association wrote legislation "which would have required the Massachusetts Rate Setting Commission to collect and publish information on individual physicians, including mortality and morbidity data and hospital discharge summaries."[51] The medical society managed to stop the legislation by persuading the governor to use his veto.

Acknowledging the strength of public opinion after another series of the *Boston Globe* articles, the medical society took the initiative and developed its own legislation designed to publicize information on a website about all physicians, including their malpractice histories, criminal convictions, and board actions. Apprised of this development, the governor and his secretary of consumer affairs and business regulation appointed an advisory committee. The governor signed the bill on August 31, 1996, but provided no additional funds to the board to develop the website or confirm the information to be posted. The Boston papers kept the board sufficiently in the news to push the medical society to develop physician profiling—a radical move that many society members vigorously protested. The informative website encouraged several other jurisdictions to follow this precedent.

When a News Series Directly Involves an Elected Official: Radical Change in Rhode Island

The linkage between news coverage and legislative action often is not direct but mediated by public outcry. The following case that appeared in the *Providence Journal* over the course of several years (1984–1986) serves as a case study of the interplay between the press, the public, and government action in effecting reform.

A Rhode Island doctor, Dr. Felix Balasco, inserted unnecessary pacemakers and monitored his patients more frequently than their conditions merited.

A reporter broke the story when she discovered that the pacemaker company was sued in Colorado federal court and that Dr. Balasco was found guilty of defrauding Medicare. The reporter's tenacity exposed a tangled story in the *Providence Journal*, starting on July 9, 1984, that entailed fraud, poor medical practice, and a regulatory system lacking necessary tools to handle such cases. There was plenty of drama involving the courts, Blue Cross's failure to alert the board, Medicare's confidentiality rules, which prohibited them from reporting to the board, and the medical board's inability to act. No one seemed to be in charge. Government agencies kept information secret, and no one did what needed to be done to protect the public.

Guilty of fraud, Dr. Balasco lost his hospital privileges. However, the medical board did not revoke his license until after the court reached its decision. Several articles provided damaging details about the board that had been re-created in 1976 in part to deal with soaring malpractice premiums. One article included the statement that unknowing patients continued to walk into this doctor's office and the story of a patient who had no money for removing an unnecessary pacemaker.[52]

On January 25, 1986, the article headline read "Prompt Action Sought in Cases of Inept, Unethical Doctors." The story integrated the demands of the legislature, the specifics of the case, and the board actions. A legislator requested a detailed account of the board activities over five years and explained that "the recent articles in the *Providence Journal* concerning the Balasco matter . . . [have] caused serious concern among members of the General Assembly." He also told the press he was looking for help on legislation to improve the disciplinary process and that his constituents were complaining about the unnecessary implants. The head of the Department of Health, according to the article, was drafting legislation to make the board more accountable and transparent and to place the board under the supervision of the department.[53]

An unprecedented public board hearing and the doctor's failure to appear brought the licensing board into the center of the story. To dramatize the story on January 30, 1986, the paper used a photograph of a patient with an unnecessary pacemaker watching the hearing. Then on February 2, 1986, an article stated that between 1978, when the board was first constituted as the current board, and 1986, they had disciplined only twenty-nine doctors. The board attorney said that the information was always public, but, according to the reporter, it was difficult to find the locked board offices. The article emphasized future changes: "The Rhode Island Department of Health is moving aggressively to transfer the board's administrative duties and offices to health department headquarters." It also said that the health director thought this move would "improve its public accessibility and accountability." The board president, a physician, also indicated he thought more board members now wished to respond to the public interest. The reporter also interviewed the executive vice president of FSMB, who explained, "The conspiracy of silence, the old boys club, has been no myth, but fortunately it is dissolving in the face of today's realities."[54]

By reiterating what state officials said they would do and claiming it was what the public wanted, the media ensured the likelihood of those changes. The president of the board indicated that while confidentially was important, the board was, in the reporter's words, "committed to publicizing disciplinary actions so the public can make informed judgments about the doctors from whom they seek care."[55] Then a February 27, 1986, article emphasized the public's concern: "It was public clamor about the matter that prompted the board to hold unprecedented public hearings in his case." The governor used the press to present legislation that would give him the authority to appoint all members and the director of the Department of Health oversight of the board. A legislator was reported as saying he was dumbfounded by board inactivity and that it had only one full time investigator while the plumbers' board had four.[56]

The Balasco story neutralized opposition to reform, and the press ensured that the governor would initiate changes by publicly reminding everyone of his promises. It limited the way the medical community could respond. The changes were radical; the board was brought under the Commissioner of Health's authority, and five of the twelve voting members had to be nonphysicians.

The press exposé tradition continued. The *Arizona Republic* published almost thirty articles from August 20 to 28, 2000, on patients victimized by negligence, doctors continuing practice after botched operations, the low rate of disciplinary actions in Arizona compared to those of other states, and the questionable practice histories of board members. The press offered enough data to buttress specific changes in the medical practice act.[57]

The Focus on Discipline

Popular media stories played up disciplinary failures; public-interest groups, government agencies, and courts continued to pay close attention to the overhaul of the medical board disciplinary process. With licensing issues largely settled, boards found more time to deal with the cases requiring disciplinary hearings, but often lacked the knowledge and tools to do so.[58]

Among the most prominent critics of the boards' failures to discipline was Dr. Sidney Wolfe. In an op-ed piece titled "Bad Doctors Get a Free Ride" in the

New York Times in 2003, Wolfe wrote: "Pennsylvania has disciplined only 5 percent of the 512 doctors who had made payments in five or more malpractice suits. . . . If medical boards, which are state agencies, are unwilling to seriously discipline doctors who repeatedly pay for malpractice including revoking medical licenses from the worst offenders—then legislators must step in and change the way the boards operate."[59]

Boards, legislatures, and medical societies paid close attention to Sidney Wolfe, whose medical credentials and leadership of Public Citizen Health Research Group, a Ralph Nader affiliate founded in 1972, were hard to ignore. Dr. Wolfe used FSMB data to rank boards according to the number of disciplinary actions per licensed doctor in each state.[60] Local newspapers often publicized the ranking and ran commentaries about the board activities around the time of the FSMB annual meetings, which were a topic of conversation, especially when Dr. Wolfe was invited to speak. The states with the highest rates enjoyed favorable publicity, while states that received poor rankings criticized the statistics. When Maryland's medical board was discussed under sunset provisions in 2001, a medical society member wrote about the proposals: "The papers have had a field day with Sidney Wolfe's criticism that based on state licensing Board's actions, Maryland ranks 40th in 1999 performance."[61] The *American Medical News* website discussed criticisms of Wolfe's rankings and quoted FSMB staff members about the measurement problems and the difficulty with interpreting Wolfe's data.[62]

Communication was not one-way in this exchange. Wolfe listened and amended his procedures. When small states complained that the narrow baseline skewed the statistics, with a handful of cases producing a wild variation in the ranking outcomes, Wolfe calculated a three-year average in 2002. As rankings kept the profession in the news, boards and legislators paid attention.

While Public Citizen focused attention on the failure to discipline errant physicians, other public-interest organizations and state agencies joined forces in producing reform. Part of this effort was in training public members, increasing the flow of data from health-care institutions, and improving the procedures for handling negligence and incompetence cases. These were the "quality of care issues" that drew the attention of a coalition for regulatory reform. The American Association of Retired People (AARP) joined the oversight reform debate, as their constituency relied heavily on medical services. The AARP leadership also realized that its local members would make good public representatives. It gave the Citizen Advocacy Center (CAC) a grant when it formed in the late 1980s to train public members of health-related boards and disseminated its views to their local associations through a pamphlet produced by the CAC. The CAC held yearly conferences for training public members, staged conferences on board issues, published a newsletter specifically addressed to public members, researched position papers on issues such as how to handle disciplinary cases, actively worked with the Office of the Inspector General (OIG) in the Department of Health and Human Services, engaged critics like Dr. Wolfe and Benjamin Shimberg, and became involved with the newly established organization for medical board administrators, Administrators in Medicine (AIM).[63] On the state level, institutes such as Center for Public Interest Law at the University of San Diego School of Law have pushed many reforms, and from 2003 to 2005, Julianne Fellmeth, the director, served as the Medical Board Enforcement Monitor in California.

The few disciplinary cases reviewed exposed problems with the procedures governing the disciplinary process. Most reports of potential problems came to the boards from patients, but many of those concerned actions over which boards had no jurisdiction, nor did they rise to the level required for action as many involved a single incident, though they often involved distasteful behavior on the part of physicians. Reports of drug abuse and sales and sexual offenses continued to rise, and boards began to take licensure actions. But most boards reviewed only a handful of negligence and incompetence cases because they were not getting reports and had insufficient tools or money at their disposal for investigation and prosecution.[64] Without improved reporting by hospitals, health maintenance organizations (HMOs), and health-care providers of "quality of care" cases, it was difficult to identify incompetent or negligent physicians—an essential step for improving patient safety. To find dangerous doctors, the medical community had to be pushed to report such cases to the boards. But then, such cases were expensive to pursue, for they required expert witnesses, protracted investigations, and lengthy hearings.[65]

Encouraged by a frustrated public and headline news stories, the OIG became involved and issued several reports on improving the disciplinary process and reporting from other health-care entities. The initial concern was spurred by the peer review organizations' failures to report problem quality-of-care cases to boards, as the OIG detailed in its first findings in *JAMA* in 1987.[66] The year before, the AMA trustees generated a report on quality of care and argued that the profession had to improve its system for disciplining its members.[67] Still, doctors wrote letters to *JAMA* criticizing the OIG report.[68] Worried that the boards did not pursue the most serious cases, the OIG and the CAC worked on parallel reports and attended each other's meetings.[69] To ensure that "good" cases entered the disciplinary process, they argued, the boards should receive reports of problem physicians from all health-care entities.[70] Most states, the OIG found, had a difficult time obtaining peer review records from hospitals, and from 1990 to 1993 about 75 percent of all hospitals never reported an incident to the National Practitioner Data Bank.[71] Another report documented case backlogs, staff shortages, renewal fees that never made it to the boards, and the limited resources that curtailed the boards' capacities to review cases.[72] The recommendations spurred some dissent from federal government agencies[73] and especially from the AMA, which "oppose[d] sharing of information" and argued that early reporting might violate due process.[74] Three public-interest groups—the AARP, the CAC, and Public Citizen—strongly supported the recommendations.[75] Only one area of consensus was reached among the organizations—funding was critical, and licensure fees should go directly to the boards.[76] Ron Wyden, chairman of the Subcommittee on Regulation, Business Opportunities, and Energy of the Committee on Small Business of the U.S. House of Representatives, supported the recommendations with legislation that failed. To help boards, the CAC created recommendations for board administrators to improve board management and legal processes.[77]

The CAC convened a conference in 1996 to discuss nonreporting to boards by health-care entities even though most states passed mandatory reporting laws. The following groups are required to report violations—hospital staff and administrators,[78] other health-care providers (HMOs, etc.)—in thirty-six states;[79] courts—in twenty states; all licensees—in thirty-six states;[80] and professional peer review organizations—in twenty-six states.[81] However, without sanctions for failure to report, many organizations find reasons to evade their obligations. This adversely affects the public interest, for without reporting, a physician who resigns under investigation, or is fired from one hospital, can move to another. In the absence of a mandatory reporting rule, doctors are encouraged to support and, perhaps, report others. The following is a sample weak call for reporting impaired or incompetent physicians to the licensing and disciplinary board: "When appropriate, an offer of personal assistance to the colleague may be the most compassionate and effective intervention. . . . Physicians also may report to the North Carolina Medical Board, and when there is no other institution reasonably likely to be able to deal with the problem, this will be the only way of discharging the duty to report."[82] Only sixteen states have the power to use civil penalties for failure to report.[83] One board used the state court to force hospitals to provide peer review records in a board's investigation of misconduct and called it "a major victory for California consumers."[84]

The Federation responded to the disciplinary issues by setting up a committee to come up with its own suggestions. "The role of the state medical board in assuring quality of care and physician competence has increasingly become a major consumer issue, and therefore has gained the interest of the federal government. . . . Two factors are necessary in order for states to successfully handle quality of care cases: (1) adequate funding and (2) a serious and ongoing commitment to protect the public interest by actively addressing quality of care cases. . . . There appears to be a public perception that state medical boards could do a better job in handling quality of care cases and assuring medical competence."[85] The Federation recognized the public as a constituency—concerned and active.

While the Federation began to see both the state and the public as active participants in the process, other medical organizations did not. An AMA and Federation dispute erupted over the involvement of medical societies in the disciplinary process. The Federation's ad hoc committee to study AMA proposals met extensively with the AMA regarding quality-of-care issues and developed a statement encouraging doctors to report unethical, impaired, and incompetent doctors to the boards and to assist boards in evaluations by serving as experts. This was not what the AMA intended; it did not enhance local societies' ability to investigate and evaluate quality-of-care cases, thus keeping the disciplinary process within the medical community, as is done in Maryland.[86]

Media attention remained an important source for generating public discussion. Reporting of problem physicians by institutions made front-page news in 2001 in the *New York Times*: "A federal program to protect patients from incompetent doctors is failing because health maintenance organizations and hospitals rarely report those doctors to the government. . . . Under federal law, H.M.O.'s and hospitals are supposed to inform the government of disciplinary actions taken against doctors for incompetence or misconduct."[87]

The Courts and the CAC: Increased Due Process

All board disciplinary actions may be subject to judicial review. Some boards felt that courts unfairly overturned their disciplinary actions or stayed sanctions of dangerous physicians while waiting years to hear a case. In 1992, the CAC produced a report that proved to be a useful guide for managing cases. Many cases raised due-process issues, but others involved the Americans with Disabilities Act, which discouraged boards from asking licensure applicants if they used drugs in the past beyond the last two years.[88]

Critically important for the operation of boards, courts require boards to grant respondents due-process rights. *Schware v. Board of Bar Examiners* in 1957 required due-process rights be given to those facing license suspension or

revocation.[89] Some boards had unresolved due-process issues in their disciplinary processes. In Arizona in 2002, a judge set aside a board decision and
remanded the case for a hearing. A doctor had been invited for an "informal
interview," but the letter had not indicated that he could have declined or
requested a full board hearing. The board panel decided that he had engaged
in "unprofessional conduct" without a formal hearing. The court ruled that the
board must inform the doctor that he had a right to a hearing, show that a
deviation from the standard of care occurred, and that the deviation resulted
in harm.[90] In other states, it is unnecessary to show actual harm, only the
potential for it. Some states avoid court challenges through consent decrees or
settlements.

Courts remain divided over burden-of-proof standards. Of the sixty-six
boards, forty-nine use "preponderance of evidence," while seventeen use the
tougher "clear and convincing" standard, making it more difficult to take licensure actions.[91] "Preponderance" is more in use and requires that the person or
persons deciding a case base the decision on the more convincing evidence,
thus, the need to establish the credibility of witnesses. "Clear and convincing"
means that persons hearing a case must believe that substantial evidence leads
to an abiding conviction of wrongdoing, which is a rather tall order. This standard may be decided in the legislature or settled in the courts upon challenge.

Moving into the Twenty-first Century

Both public members and doctors who joined boards in the 1970s and 1980s
describe them as short-staffed and disorganized. Those who remember the old
days describe the twenty-first-century boards as models of efficiency by comparison. A retired doctor who worked with the attorney general's office on
disciplinary cases told me what it was like under the old system, when a
staff member would address the board, "Here are thirty cases about which perhaps something should be done." The board would answer, "Here are the fifteen about which you should be concerned." The lawyers would chime in,
"These are the two we can handle given the resources." A public member serving in the early 1980s on a medical board of a large state described the boxes
of unanswered complaints she found when she was, in her words, "drafted"
onto the board.[92]

Boards paid attention to local constituencies and often ignored national
trends. Some operated in a democratic fashion and strove for transparency;
others concentrated power in the hands of the profession and shielded operations from the public. Since legislatures authorized medical boards, the latter did
not sit entirely within civil society, but some worked entirely independently

from the state. Others sat within the state bureaucracies. This reflected in part local political cultures, the interest that the public took in local governance, and the responsiveness of legislators to their constituents.

Despite years of struggle to add public members to boards, three states in 2011 did not have voting public members: Alabama, Louisiana, and Mississippi. States that added public members at a late date often faced resistance from the board and medical societies. In 1992 the Tennessee board president repeated a position first articulated three decades earlier: "The issues with which the Board of Medical Examiners must deal are more often than not beyond the ability of a public member to understand due to the scientific nature of the issues."[93] Alabama partially relented in 1995 when it added a public member on its appeals board, but its medical board remained free of public representation. Six states added public members for the first time before 1975, twenty-two between 1975 and 1979, ten between 1980 and 1984, six between 1985 and 1989, and three after 1990.[94]

It took time for public members to carve out a niche for themselves, with several gaining positions as board officers, including the 1997 FMSB president, Susan Spaulding, who wrote, "In a short time, public members began chairing medical boards, showing public and professional members [sitting] on medical boards shoulder to shoulder doing the same thing—protecting the public."[95] She continues to be active and supports many public members in their efforts, but sometimes public members have maintained a silent presence on their boards.

The percentage of public members is about one-quarter on most boards, but on seven boards public members make up a third or more. As a rule, governors appoint both medical and public members, but often choose doctors from medical society lists. Some public members appear to be appointed because of their political contributions, but most have been sufficiently active to come to the attention of the governor and are college graduates.[96] Most serve for no more than two terms of three or four years each and often feel they have insufficient training and direction. The Citizen Advocacy Center maintains a public member network and organizes a yearly training meeting, but only a handful of public members attend CAC conferences as boards lack resources to send them. When the CAC offered to pay for attendance, few accepted. Those who attend meetings report learning a good deal about their roles and the issues facing boards.[97] Only a few public members attend the Federation annual meeting or maintain affiliation with state-level public-interest groups. Most learning, we have to assume, occurs through local board member interactions.

Transparency has improved. In the 1970s boards worked largely in isolation from each other and the public. Boards are now more open to exchanging information and providing information to the public. Several sources of information on disciplined physicians are currently available, and some meetings and disciplinary procedures are public. All states have websites where one can usually find a list of doctors sanctioned by the board, a list of open meetings, and information about the board organization and medical practice acts. In some states, all physicians are listed with their specialties, board actions against them, and settled malpractice cases. Each state has its own way of presenting the data, deciding which data should be made publicly available and when. If a physician is found to have committed misconduct, some states put the entire disciplinary opinion on the site, while others include only the final disposition. In 2002 Dr. Wolfe ranked the quality of the websites maintained by the boards for the first time.[98]

Since 1985, a greater volume of national disciplinary data has become available.[99] The publicly available Federation Board Action Data Bank engendered much less hostility from medical organizations than the National Practitioner Data Bank (NPDB), developed by the Public Health Service, which lists all licensure actions, malpractice suits, and suspensions of hospital privileges but is open only to health-care entities and licensing boards. In 1993, the AMA House of Delegates voted for the dissolution of the NPDB.[100] But Representative Ron Wyden of Oregon sought to make the NPDB public as a way of enhancing "consumer choice."[101] Dr. Sidney Wolfe and Anne Paxton of *ProForum* supported the opening of the data bank. Wolfe complained that as a physician he did not have access to the data that he needed to make wise referrals and that patients could use to make informed decisions.[102] According to Paxton, in weighing the public interest over the right to privacy, she opted to make the information public.[103]

The Freedom of Information Act served to help open meetings in most states, but boards differ in the kinds of proceedings they open to the public. Some have special public meetings, others convene open disciplinary hearings, and still others hold open discussions of the final disciplinary orders. The timing of making the process public varies as well. In some states nothing is public until the results are final and only then if the charges are upheld. To examine variation in transparency, I used the FSMB data from the Federation Exchange to calculate an index of transparency that tracks the distribution of materials to the public and other boards.[104] The index shows a good deal of variation among the states in disseminating information to the public and exchanging information with other boards. More boards are clustered toward the low transparency pole (16 boards) than the high (9 boards).[105] The patterns shift continuously as boards make decisions and legislators make changes.

A major shift during the last two decades of the twentieth century increased the links between some boards and state bureaucracies. Legislation moved some further into state bureaucracies, while other boards evolved through internal growth and influence of staff and members.[106] On one end of this spectrum, *state boards*, government employees make at least some decisions, and board employees largely work for the state (ten boards). At the other end, twenty-four *independent boards* collect all their fees, set their own budgets, hire and fire staff, have members nominated only from the medical society's list, make their own policies, and issue position papers. Thirty-two *mixed boards* fall in between, with the state and the board each providing employees and with varying rights to evaluate, hire, and fire staff.[107] The balance shifts continuously. These variations affect, but do not determine, the manner in which boards function. Although most boards make disciplinary and licensing decisions, staff, formally or informally, influence the progress of cases through the system. Although discipline has increased and boards look more to the public to establish their goals, the medical societies maintain a hold on many boards, particularly those independent from the state.

Increasing Struggle: The Medical Societies Are Not the Only Constituency

As the number of groups interested in board work increased, boards and medical societies began to acknowledge different interests. Medical societies, even when they acknowledged a need for improvement, wanted boards to remain focused on the medical community. But many boards are becoming organizations increasingly oriented toward the public. Most boards recognize that their goals and constituencies are different from those of the medical societies. However, the willingness to proceed against the wishes of medical societies varies, as do the boards' abilities to do so. Even at the state-embedded extreme, the medical societies have influence over changes in medical practice acts through their lobbyists and also influence board member selection. The links between boards and local medical societies range from indirect—"it is difficult for us to do this when the medical society will oppose it"—to direct connections, like those observed in the state of Maryland, where a peer review committee appointed by the medical society reviewed quality-of-care complaints.[108]

It takes time for a board and medical society to develop separate identities. For instance, in Michigan the board was concerned about the increasing authority of the state, its president arguing in a 1978 interview: "This is a job that has to be done and it is best that it be done by physicians. If we turn it over to others, we are in trouble."[109] To him the board was a medical organization. Two years later, Dr. H. M. Andre, a medical society member, criticized the changes concerning continuing medical education that the board struggled to enact, saying, "It is high time we in the medical profession educate the public that our profession as a whole is providing quality care at a reasonable cost, and that we are being burdened with restrictions imposed by the government."[110]

By 1986, R. W. Hood, director of the Michigan Department of Licensing and Regulation under whose authority the board worked, wrote in the medical society journal: "[We] continually rethink our process. How can we be more responsive to consumers? How can we better serve our licensees? How can we maximize our resources?"[111] The idea to publish an article about protecting the public came two years later when Judy Marr wrote in the medical society journal, "Both Doctor Vincent [board member] and new board administrator Thomas J. DeKornfeld, MD, emphasize that it is the board's job to protect the public, not to protect physicians."[112] Despite this greater sensitivity toward the need for transparency, some local medical associations continued to lobby for taking control away from the boards. One proposal encouraged medical societies to become officially involved with the regulatory process. In 1988 Dr. J. K. Baum, president of the Washtenau County (Michigan) Medical Society, wrote, "Perhaps the board's functions and even the board itself should be run by the State Medical Society."[113] But Michigan increased its public members from 21 percent in 1978 to 42 percent in 1994.[114]

In New Jersey, acknowledgment that consumers and the state were active players came earlier than in many other states. In 1971, New Jersey doctors sounded the alarm about state encroachment on their territory: "The State Boards are forced to follow political directives instead of accepted Medical opinion. . . . The public has to look to the professional expertise in its professional societies and medical schools, rather than to legislators, in order to develop programs for the delivery of a satisfactory program for health care and for its protection."[115] But in 1979, Dr. Joseph Riggs, executive director of the New Jersey Board, acknowledged that, with the addition of two public members, the board's performance improved: "This is a conscientious and diligent Board, consumer oriented. . . . The Medical Society of New Jersey should be congratulated for having the wisdom to plan a conference about medical discipline."[116] The need to keep an arm's-length relationship between boards and medical societies is hard to overstate. Dr. F. J. Malta, a board member, took pains to emphasize that the board was charged with protecting the health, safety, and welfare of consumers and had the power to police.[117] The link between the state medical societies and the boards must remain problematic but not adversarial, according to Dr. Sanford Lewis. The relations should be "friendly antagonistic," with the two organizations engaged in constructive debates: "Let the societies represent medicine's 'ego,' with the boards, appropriately, characterized as the 'superego.'"[118]

Each state had to wage its own struggle to establish separate society and board identities. Sometimes change came when a state board member, active in the Federation, took a political stand. Dr. G. J. Carroll, a member of the Virginia board, hailed the defeat of Virginia House Bill 454, which required continuing medical education, and the defeat of another bill that would have added two citizen members to the board of medicine in 1979.[119] But in 1987 Dr. Gerald Bechamps, president of the board and later president of the Federation, wrote: "Until recently, we have been unresponsive to the need for public protection. . . . [We will cooperate] with the Governor's office in supporting the addition of two public members to the Board to enhance public accountability. . . . We look forward to new and innovative ideas and continuing cooperation with government officers, legislators, and agencies to demonstrate to the public that we are responsive to their needs and demands."[120]

Nowadays, board members often differ in their outlook on pressing issues from their colleagues in the medical society. One medical member of an independent board explained the relationship to me this way: "It is important to maintain a tension between the medical society and the board. We need to have a relationship with the medical society, as we could not get new legislation without their help." When asked if they were ever on opposite sides of legislative issues, he replied "yes," using a dispute over continuing medical education as the case in point. He thought that the legislation would go through, but the medical society defeated most of the changes with massive lobbying efforts. Independent boards differentiate themselves from medical societies, but maintaining distance is a continuous struggle.

Most of the relationships between boards and societies are informal; societies use their resources, lobbyists, and informal ties. Even boards under state bureaucracies must deal with medical societies on legislative issues. In one instance, commenting on pending legislation designed to weaken the disciplinary process, a board member used the expression "we believe," his reference to "we" indicating that he did not separate his function on the board from his membership in the medical society. The proposed changes would make the investigatory process overly cumbersome and so heavily slanted toward physicians that disciplinary actions would be hard to achieve.

Trade-offs are common, and indeed necessary, for achieving a board's agenda. Negotiations with medical societies take place when boards try to take legislative action to increase their jurisdiction over physicians. The medical practice act in Virginia lowered the bar for a charge of misconduct. The board's executive director, a physician, explained, "The medical society of Virginia accepts the change. That's because the legislation calls for a 'confidential consent agreement' between the board and the doctor instead of public discipline in cases involving minor misconduct with little or no injury to the patient or the public. . . . The changes were initiated by a state audit and news stories about problem doctors practicing without losing licenses. The public outcry led legislators to change the practice act and the medical society worked on the proposals."[121] Even when board members are fully aware of the need to maintain a separate identity, they know they have to continue working with medical societies.

Medical societies tend to look at issues from the perspective of physicians. They are particularly concerned with scope-of-practice issues—that is, bills permitting other health-related professions to perform functions traditionally reserved for physicians. Under the headline "Physicians Win Big in States over Scope of Practice Issues," Jay Greene wrote in an AMA online journal, "The 2001 state legislature sessions proved a banner year for physicians as they defeated a slew of scope of practice bills that sought to give additional independent practice rights to advanced-practice nurses . . . physicians scored well. . . . They found success with strategies that linked grass roots lobbying with collaborative efforts between state medical associations, specialty societies and the AMA. . . . The theme was educational difference between physicians and nonphysicians."[122] Several years earlier, however, the medical board in one state chose to work with the nursing board against the medical society and passed legislation to permit the independent practice of advanced practice nurses. Independent practice for nurse practitioners passed in many states. And in New Mexico, over the medical society's protests, legislation was passed on March 6, 2002, allowing psychologists with additional training to prescribe some medications.

By 2000, few states allowed medical societies official board functions. The Maryland board, however, had a close relationship to the medical society, despite working under the state bureaucracy with state-employed staff with some decision-making responsibilities. Maryland gave the medical society official status in 1976. Dr. J. I. Berman, chair of the medical society committee that evaluated board cases, explained the new act: "There was considerable frustration about the fact that the Medical Society itself had no statutory recognition in the old law and thus no defined role in dealing with physicians practicing badly. . . . We are faced with the need to protect the physician's rights as he appears before the medical society's committees and the need to maintain the usually close peer relationships. . . . Our statute, with all its problems, has provided organized medicine in Maryland with the opportunity to police itself and to meaningfully assure the public that only competent physicians may practice."[123]

That same year Dr. J. J. Coller, chair of the commission on medical discipline, wrote: "The local committees of the Medical Society see themselves as fatherly, advising and educational bodies—and so it should be. . . . The Commission sees its role as one of protection, not punishment. It attempts to protect all citizens of the state, including physicians. . . . It is not necessary to revoke numerous licenses to set examples."[124] As we can see, the constituency in Maryland is the physician, not the public. More than ten years later, the medical society still worried the board might get too close to its impaired physicians committee: "The welfare of society and the welfare of the individual impaired physician are inseparable." A public report, according to this writer, "conspicuously misinterpreted and misrepresented [cases] to create a 'public outcry' for mandatory reporting to the State Board."[125]

Despite criticism from the public and state, the Maryland medical society maintained its official role according to *News and Views* of the CAC.[126] The health secretary warned the board its relationship was too close to the medical society after an article in the *Baltimore Sun* exposed a physician with eighteen malpractice cases and no medical board record, even though regulations required investigation of a doctor with three or more malpractice cases. Allegations of substandard care were referred to two medical society members to investigate, with a proviso that it was up to them to decide whether the board should get involved. Maryland ranked among the lowest states in taking serious disciplinary actions during the prior five years. Legislators also objected to the medical society's role in the regulatory process. The CAC opposed the "blanket amnesty to practitioners simply for reporting an error, regardless of its gravity and consequences."[127]

In February 2002, the Maryland legislature proposed a statute to separate the medical society and board, but the proposal failed.[128] The proposal included repealing provisions requiring ten members to be selected from the medical society's list, eliminating the requirement that the medical society conduct investigations, and mandating a list of physician disciplinary actions on the website. According to the CAC, it was a wasted opportunity not to add more public members. But Thomas Allen, MD, chair of the MedChi

(Maryland Medical Society) Task Force on Medical Discipline and Quality Assurance committee, argued that the board's "prevailing philosophy should be nonpunitive in nature . . . to formulate interventions for corrective action . . . would not be discipline, and would be confidential and non-discoverable . . . establishing specifically that an individual adverse event could not become the basis for a sanction if it is reported voluntarily."[129]

The Maryland medical society succeeded in keeping the board a more "medical" than public organization. As in almost 30 percent of states, the medical society was the sole source of nominations of medical members.[130] Informally, doctors can, and sometimes do, put pressure on individual board members to take particular positions. Some board members may even receive calls from colleagues to get involved with disciplinary cases and policy issues. In one state, several of the doctors on the board were former state medical society presidents. While open attempts to influence the outcome in particular cases are probably rare, direct pressure was applied in a few cases I observed. In one, a physician's general support of "public protection" and public members changed in the face of pressure from colleagues in the medical society on a matter of medical society–initiated board policy that would have made public members second-class. Although he had been against the medical society's position, this physician made a strong argument supporting the medical society. His increasing reliance on referrals from other physicians may have changed his mind.

Resolving Issues in the Twenty-First Century

Three licensing issues concerned boards at the turn of the twenty-first century—how to facilitate interstate portability of licenses, how to implement a new clinical competency exam, and how to ensure and evaluate a physician's competency over a medical career. Each issue was discussed in terms of the public interest by the broader public. In each case, the Federation and the AMA took different positions. In some instances, the Federation moved closer to the position of public-interest groups and away from medical societies. Pew, a private foundation, issued two major reports in 1995 through its Pew Health Professions Commission that met with strong objections from the medical community but greatly stimulated the discussion of licensing in the late 1990s. Only the new clinical competency exam issue was resolved; it did not require state action.

The Pew Health Professions Commission reports, dealing with the reform of health-care regulation, were "Reforming Health Care Workforce Regulation" and "Critical Challenges: Revitalizing the Health Professions for the Twenty-First

Century." Membership on the task force for the second report included members of the CAC, and Pew staff attended several CAC meetings.[131] The Federation withheld its support for the recommendations on the grounds that the reports failed to give the medical community enough credit for the changes it had already made. The plan, regulatory overhaul, was revolutionary rather than evolutionary in nature, the medical profession concluded.[132] The reports echoed the concerns raised by the DOL and HEW that pointed to the absence of licensing uniformity across states,[133] the lack of public accountability of boards, unresolved scope of practice issues, the lack of public protection, and the difficulty of obtaining information about disciplinary outcomes.[134] The report also called for the evaluation of board performance, the provision of resources to develop cost-effective and uniform disciplinary measures, and the development of tools for assessing continuing competency of practicing physicians.[135] This last suggestion became central.

One issue that riled the medical licensing community was Pew's support of federal licensure requirements in light of telemedicine and its need for license portability. The Federation argued in 1995 that state licensure facilitated variation in local needs; however, standardization would facilitate what technology offers—treating people across state borders. Playing on fears of federal involvement, the executive vice president of FSMB stressed that, if they did not develop uniform standards, federal licensure was possible.[136] To facilitate licensure the Federation opened a credentialing data bank in 2002 centralizing the verifications necessary for licensing and developed a streamlined model license application for telemedicine. However, despite the AMA's dislike of federal involvement, it worked against the FSMB proposal for a special license to practice telemedicine. The president of the Federation, writing in 1996 in the *Federation Bulletin*, explained: "The House of Delegates [of the Federation] adopted as policy . . . physicians who wished to practice telemedicine across state lines to have a special license. . . . AMA adopted as policy at their June 1996 Annual Meeting that any physician practicing telemedicine across state lines is required to have a full and unrestricted license in the state where the patient resides. I fear that opposite policies by two great organizations will create an adversarial relationship between licensure boards and state medical associations . . . I see trouble ahead!"[137]

Continuing competency, specifically maintenance of licensure, was actively considered by boards and the Federation but opposed by some medical groups. In 2003, the Federation established the Special Committee on the Maintenance of Licensure, and a staff member of the Federation, Frances Cain, reviewed boards' efforts to measure or ensure continuing competency as a response to the Pew reports and the Institute of Medicine.[138] California started discussions of recertification but tabled the measure because of cost. The Nevada board stepped back from implementing a pilot study of time-limited licensure when the board membership changed. The Texas board in 2002 planned to ask the legislature to require proficiency testing of physicians every ten years, but *American Medical News* reported that the medical society opposed the changes, saying that "the leadership of the Texas Medical Association is not sold on the legislation."[139] The Federation established summits and brought together a diverse group of medical organizations, public-interest groups, and government players.[140] Little has been achieved yet, but it is a growing topic of discussion by public-interest groups, the FSMB, and other medical organizations. This issue will take some time to settle as it involves the coordination of so many different interests and will require local affirmation. Several states intend to begin requirements for relicensure.

In 2002, the new entry-level examination for license applicants to demonstrate clinical and communication skills divided the Federation and AMA.[141] The Federation voted to support such an exam in 1999, but the AMA objected to it, supporting a resolution in its House of Delegates in December 2001 brought by medical students that proposed that the NBME reconsider its plans. The medical students threatened to withdraw from the AMA if the AMA supported it. The AMA expected protests at the 2003 Federation meeting, but none materialized. Limited protests took place on the state level. *American Medical News* printed articles, one entitled "AMA against NBME's Clinical Skills Test," and a second, a year later, "AMA Takes Aim at Skills Exam."[142] The articles also highlighted public demand for improved interpersonal skills and the belief that poor communication increased medical errors. The exam was given first in 2004.

Conversely, implementation of policies that require local change is a struggle, requiring strong public voices and legislative debate. Boards remain responsive to the different local environments. A newsletter article addressing California physicians in 2008 stated, "California continues to be interested in and supportive of facilitating the benefits of national licensure ... but before that commitment can be made, California must ensure that its criteria are met."[143]

As medical organizations developed different interests, so did citizen and public-interest groups. For example, in 2006, Republican Governor George Pataki of New York vetoed a bill proposed by a citizen's group that would have hamstrung the New York medical board's disciplinary process by making legal procedures to revoke a license more complex. A patient advocacy group, angry with the board for sanctioning physicians whom they supported, proposed the changes. The state medical society, several specialty groups, the ALJ association, the FSMB, the New York Department of Health, and several patient advocacy groups also opposed the legislation. Boards are now more critically observed not only by the local medical society but also by public-interest groups, the state, and the press.

Chapter 5

Rhetorics of Law, Medicine, and Public Interest Shape Board Work

The language of public protection slowly crept into board work, but it is still often overwhelmed by the discourses of medicine and law in shaping deliberations. The language of "protecting the public" began to appear regularly in the *Federation Bulletin* in the 1970s and was heard increasingly at Federation meetings. While no longer silenced, the voices of public members are often muffled, their votes sometimes fail to make a difference, and their role in board deliberations remains ambiguous—all of these problems reflect the difficulty of connecting with public constituencies.[1] Some critics insist that nothing much can be done to alter this situation, given the logistics of mobilizing public opinion and articulating public good. Some still do not think that public members belong on boards, as a nonphysician critic of the British General Medical Council argued in 1994: "Where issues are raised during the course of proceedings which require the application of medical training or expertise in their determination, it seems that the presence of lay members could result in the decision-making being flawed. . . . It would not seriously detract from the accountability of the profession for lay members to be removed."[2] However, this view is overly pessimistic; it fails to acknowledge the extent to which board members are open to sensible arguments and can be engaged in democratic deliberations undistorted by vested interests and blatant self-seeking and that cases often involve moral and character decisions, are not highly "technical," and are well within the competence of an educated person. Medical and legal discourses also provide narrative structures that open some venues for discussion while closing others, notably those central to public protection.

The language of the public/civic sphere is distinct from medical discourse. It tends to be less developed and less articulated than its medical counterpart and typically comes into play at the final stage of the disciplinary process. The weakness of the public domain discourse affects both public members and physicians—all board members stand to learn about its intricacies. Hence, the importance of educating all board members remains about patients' needs.

The more deliberations focus on disciplinary issues, the greater role the legal and administrative language assumes in board deliberations.[3] Law can provide a strong narrative structure for disciplinary cases, and administrative efficiency shapes the process as the volume of cases facing boards grows while resources do not. Understanding the peculiarities of legal and administrative discourse is all the more important since administrators and lawyers increasingly act as gatekeepers making decisions, shaping board agendas and talk, and influencing what comes before the board.

Boards collectively develop ways of doing and talking about work that are sometimes difficult to change. As we have seen in earlier chapters, boards were historically medical organizations linked to medical societies and communities. Medical discourse, for most physicians, is a habit, a default position on which they fall—unless pushed to do otherwise. The public/civic domain, by contrast, is less of a "habit" for most participants, is often vague, and requires effort to decipher how a public "might" think. Administrative staff and lawyers bring their own frames of talk to board meetings that provide a counterbalance to the medical discursive domain.[4]

The balance of discourses varies among boards, but once a given discourse emerges as dominant in a discussion, it opens certain avenues for questioning and invites a particular kind of evidence. Public and medically trained members come to the board armed with favorite discursive modes, yet they are not inexorably tied to their ways of talking—most board members are open to sensible arguments, but professional roles are important, especially for lawyers and doctors. The ability to listen, question, persuade, and take the role of the other are essential as well.

Interest-group political theory is built around the assumption that humans know their interests and are bent on profit maximizing. "Rational choice" actors are driven by egoistic, self-serving agendas rather than by irrational values like altruism.[5] From this angle, physicians have little incentive to expose bad doctors in their midst, for this would tarnish the prestige of the medical profession and make it difficult for physicians to maintain professional autonomy. The interest-group perspective casts the public as a monolithic group composed of like-minded individuals who have its interest represented by public members.[6] Appeals to common good and justice are regarded with jaundiced eyes. If this model were right, then physicians would prevail, their majority position on the board assuring success for their shared agenda. Reality does not support this conclusion. The public and profession are not always at loggerheads; neither doctors nor public members necessarily vote as monolithic blocks; and each side is capable of taking the perspective of the other. After all, physicians are members of the public who have family members vulnerable to unscrupulous physicians, just as public members see respectable doctors in their private lives. "Protecting the public interest" and "in the interest of the profession" are phrases that conceal more specific frames for interpreting issues and cases. We should not forget, also, that both professional and public interests are often fragmented, with doctors holding conflicting agendas and public members bringing to the board different beliefs and experiences.

What is more important for physicians—to lower the malpractice insurance rates by weeding out bad physicians or to hide poor physicians damaging the profession's reputation? One physician active for many years in the Federation said, "Get rid of the bad guys—it's making us look bad." His colleague concurred, saying, "They dirty it for others." These judgments were couched in the language of the medical profession, yet they are quite different in substance and inconsistent with protecting their own. The real world is more muddled than interest-group politics allow. Certain policies or decisions may divide medical specialties. Some are uneasy about independent practice and prescription-writing privileges for nurse practitioners, claiming that such nurses endanger the public, particularly when nurses take over procedures that fall within the scope of practice of their specialty. Doctors may see such an extension as a threat to their income and status while hiding their pecuniary interests under the "protect the public" rhetoric. Others frame it as public access to services. Doctors outside the specialty are more likely to conclude that nurses operate safely and increase access to health care. On one board, the physicians were divided on this issue, with the surgeons less concerned about advanced practice nurses working independently than family practice physicians and internists on whose "turf" nurses would be treading. It is difficult for public members to take a stance in such cases, to know which argument has greater merit—increasing safety or maximizing access. But divisions within the ranks of the professionals and the public presence create a possibility for the articulation of diverse perspectives in the decision-making process. In one case, when board physicians reached a consensus that nurse practitioners could work independently because of their education, they were challenged unsuccessfully by the medical society.[7] Although professionals may have conflicting interests, doctors come to board work with common language, relationships, experiences, and evaluation techniques.

The "public interest" is also internally divided, sometimes pitting one group of patients against another. Some patients of doctors involved in sexual misconduct cases were perfectly satisfied with the physicians' medical services and unimpressed by sexual misconduct charges. In one case, the attorney general, an elected official, was caught between two public constituencies, each urging him to make a different decision. Wishing to avoid an appeal, he settled for a minor sanction. Another case involved an internist who treated patients in a poor rural area with few specialists and followed patients for many years. According to a specialist's testimony, this practitioner had not been doing an adequate job in a specialty area. A question emerged—is it better to hold the generalist to a specialist's standards, revoke the license and let patients go without treatment, or to let an internist lacking in a specialized training continue offering medical help in this underserved region? There is more than one way to define the public interest.

Despite conflicts among specialties and types of practices, medical members and staff have similar styles of education and experiences.[8] Public members enter as volunteers but are often not well practiced in articulating the public interest, even though they all have families, neighbors, and coworkers who share their concerns. Physicians are accustomed to self-regulation, and boards have traditionally been their turf. Also, they are taught and teach others how to practice medicine and how to deal with their own and others' mistakes. Lawyers are trained in legal language and procedures and are backed or challenged by courts. Public members have an affinity with civic groups, legislatures, and their own work associations. Most public members are not linked to physicians or health-care institutions because of the way most state statutes define them. As early as the late 1970s, consumer groups expressed their concerns about the qualifications of consumer members.[9]

Medical/Professional Discursive Domain

Most doctors know what it is like to be evaluated and evaluate others, and they know that physicians make errors.[10] Young physicians learn to talk about errors they make, both among themselves and through criticisms by supervising physicians; this experience shapes their working habits. Hospital rounds also train doctors to present cases and develop an account of illnesses.[11] These narratives have a conventional structure and content, in which "the case" is the basic unit of thought. These presentations are not the patients' stories, but the medical construction of them. Students become accustomed to particular orderings of stories, evidence assessment, and filling in gaps with anecdotes to create bridges between general rules of disease and particular facts of an illness.[12] This is what doctors are familiar with, what they often rely on in constructing disciplinary cases.

Many doctors see their world as filled with uncertainty.[13] For example, in graduate medical training, internal medicine residents and interns learn to define and avoid common medical errors.[14] "That could be me" is the way Dr. Atul Gawande explained doctors' reactions after hearing about errors.[15] They learn to deal with unanticipated negative consequences of medical interventions that may increase morbidity or pain. In striving to develop competency and confidence, doctors make errors and learn to use strategies to explain problems away through commonplace expressions like "medicine is as much an art as a science," "no right or wrong exists," or "only differences of opinion exist." Physicians do admit error but often learn to shift blame elsewhere, charging a system error or the patient's failure to follow directions. They also learn to narrow the definition of mistakes by saying that what they did was inconsequential, that someone reversed their error, that everyone makes mistakes, that no one died, or that it couldn't be helped. Subordinates during surgical residencies receive a confrontational "talking-to" by supervisors particularly for normative errors, such as the failure to follow established routines, which suggests lack of competence and could result in losing one's position.[16] The patients, doctors learn, have no input in their evaluation, nor do hospital administrators, who can only second-guess the doctors' clinical judgments. Doctors learn to feel accountable to their peers, and anticipating their colleagues' judgment becomes a habit they fall back on when evaluating board disciplinary cases.

Grand rounds for presenting unexpected successes and morbidity and mortality (M&M) conferences for discussing "mistakes" or unexpected failures are models of evaluation and are educational.[17] During an M&M discussion about error, the presenting doctor "puts on the hair shirt," admitting error and explaining publicly what he or she learned from it so that others can benefit from the experience. The goal is to learn from complications, modify actions and judgments based on experience, and prevent recurrence of costly mistakes. The analysis of why mistakes happen takes precedence, and no formal sanctions result.[18] Cases in internal medicine conferences are chosen largely because of their teaching value, not because of the significance of the medical error.[19] As Dr. Gawande observed, "The successful M&M presentation inevitably involves a certain elision of detail and a lot of passive verbs."[20]

They both discourage self-doubt and foster denial. All physicians in residency programs have experience with such events, and they continue to draw on this experience.

Credentialing and peer review are occasions when physicians' records are evaluated in a hospital setting, but such occasions are infrequent and rarely result in formal sanctions. Credentialing generally involves examining the educational and training records for hospital privileges. Peer review by a hospital's staff may result in the loss of some privileges. If privileges are denied or severely limited, the loss must be reported to the National Practitioner Data Bank (NPDB) and, in most states, to the licensing board.[21] But the deliberations and records are often privileged from judicial disclosure.[22] Many times the outcome is some form of remediation—either retraining or supervision of a particular task. Sometimes a physician will "read the writing on the wall," leave the hospital, and move to a different one before official sanctions are applied. Most infractions by students and residents lead to permission to remain in the system, even if the young doctors are dismissed from a particular residency program. Many physician board members have participated in such discussions.

All board members have to evaluate the practice of medicine. Since 1999, roughly 12 percent of disciplinary cases nationally that resulted in sanctions included violations that required technical knowledge to evaluate, meaning that most cases could be understood by a non-physician.[23] Even cases of negligence and incompetence sometimes do not require complicated technical knowledge to evaluate and also involve ethical issues. Public members do need to develop a level of understanding of what happened and what the standards of care are in these cases. Medical professionals sometimes take positions that nonphysicians cannot readily understand. Debates continue among social scientists and philosophers, with some contending that the difference is unbridgeable and others insisting that the skill gap is exaggerated, that the lines separating scientists and the public are far from bright. Harry Collins and Robert Evans argue that those insisting on the gap between expert and nonexpert knowledge are engaged in power play. They distinguish between contributory and interactional forms of expertise, with the former involving actors who participate in the growth of knowledge and the latter implying the ability to use knowledge and communicate well.[24] In their roles as disciplinary decision makers, neither physicians nor public members need or use contributory knowledge.[25] Physicians are asked to provide the standard of care and assess whether a physician has met it. Public members are not asked to opine on the standard of care, but they need to understand the standard and what actually

happened to weigh in on decisions about complicated diagnoses and treatment. Few public members can ask very specific medical questions or feel confident whether a medical error was avoidable without substantial discussion.
But if malpractice juries are capable of informed judgment when given proper
instructions, so are public members on medical boards who are also well educated and repeat players, unlike many jurors.[26] Once the standards and evidence are explained to them, public members can assess whether a particular
diagnosis or treatment failed to meet standards of care. Note that physicians
also require explanations as to a standard of care in areas beyond their
specialties. Public members need—and have the right to expect—expert advice
and explication of facts, which will allow them to participate in board
deliberations and contribute to decisions.

The evaluation and remediation process with which all doctors are familiar sensitizes them to a particular kind of narrative that is rich in stories about
the problem doctor's status, character, professional history, and standing in the
community. Several administrators told me that physician board members felt
comfortable talking to the physicians facing the board about their wrongful
actions and their possible causes and that they saw educational value in such
exercises, which they preferred to formal hearings and sitting in judgment. As
board members develop "understanding" of problems, they form an opinion
about the problem physician's readiness to change.[27] This is not a highly
technical exercise or one physicians have been particularly trained for. What
they strive for is understanding and remediation, just as they do at M&M
conferences, where colleagues sit in judgment. This is how the Texas medical
board secretary framed the issue for the medical society magazine: "Dr. Spires
pointed out that the board is rehabilitative rather than punitive in nature.
When a license is ordered to be suspended, revoked or cancelled, the Board
may, by majority vote, 'probate' the order and require the physician to conform
to certain conditions . . . to correct the problems leading to the violation."[28]
This statement was made in 1972, but about twenty years later a speaker at the
Federation annual meeting concurred, "We have failed when we have to resort
to revocation. I don't like body counts." "We reserve discipline for the
physician who has already hurt someone," another board member observed,
"treatment is better because what is best is that the doctor needs to make a
living. We have invested so much in him, it would be wrong to throw it away."
A medical director explained to me why he thought doctors were so interested
in the problem physicians' perspectives: "The news media sees 'protecting
the public' as the investigation and prosecution of doctors with little regard for
the doctor's perspective."

It is not uncommon for public members to adopt the mindset that rehabilitation should be the board's principal goal. At one Federation meeting, a public member explained to me that a physician found guilty in a malpractice suit had already been punished and should be rehabilitated by the board. We "pamper with impairment," as he put it. The question of public protection does not figure in this discourse. I heard public members talking about the "peer review" of the board as though they were entirely outside the process. One explained to a group of public members that regulation is "too intrusive—we need a kinder, gentler approach. We need to save the doctor." Another saw her role on the board in this way:

> My contributions to the Health Professions Committee—we stipulate doctors under court order for chemical dependency or bipolar—[it is] not a public order—so when the numbers come out we are very low [a reference to Sidney Wolfe's ranking], and it doesn't take into account that we have many in this program. They are monitored because we are a rehab state and doctors do it voluntarily, which if it were public, they wouldn't come forward because it would embarrass their families and associates. It is completely confidential, and we are protecting the public and yet we are concerned with the doctor too.

This state also sent sexual offenders to a rehabilitation program. An investigator from the same board told me that, since it takes so long to educate a doctor, it was best to salvage them from their addictions and let sex offenders practice with chaperones after treatment. Staff, hired by the board in this state, concurred with the rehabilitation philosophy.

Some public members changed their position on rehabilitation as the only legitimate approach after attending a public members' meeting: "Our contention is that the docs on our board want to rehabilitate. Maybe it's a new thing but in [our state] it has been for years and years. Everyone is asked to rehabilitate themselves but recently I said, 'Isn't there a time limit?' He [the doctor] goes on and on and keeps coming back to the board. Isn't there supposed to be a time limit or how many times can they come back?" Another public member at the same meeting explained the rehabilitative policies of her board that she questioned:

> We have this tough case because forty-three cases came to light, and we did a temporary suspension. . . . There is another contested case, and this is such a mess. . . . I've never heard of this when we have a contested case and three new cases came to light, . . . the ALJ presided

over one case but not over the other cases—what do we do? It was doctors versus public members. How can we agree to a stipulation to an order when we don't know about the other cases? This is the third review committee that has come forward with a stipulation, and he has been allowed to practice for ten years without any supervision. He goes on and on, and the board says that he failed to do what he was supposed to do, and he comes up before the board, and then they said he did this much, and they say he can continue with supervision eight to ten years. They think he can be rehabilitated?

In response to the complaints about boards being too rehabilitative, a public member explained how his board tried to move away from the rehabilitative model. "Initially when we started our retraining program we found out that only a small percentage of the physicians could be retrained. We were instructed to think about whether the physician had insight into the problem, knew what he has done wrong and that it was wrong, and, second, are they motivated to getting retrained? Is this doctor someone who has been bucking you the whole way, or is he interested in being retrained?" This member still talked in the language of medicine that emphasizes understanding and not the language of public good that favors patient's safety. Rehabilitation focuses on the physician, rather than the patients, with the guiding question, "Does he understand what he has done and how to correct the error of his ways?" A practicing lawyer serving as a public member qualified his commitment to rehabilitation with a "whenever possible" rider:

> The public member becomes the 'social conscience' of the boards. . . . Standards are invariably determined by the health care providers themselves. Thus, it is not unreasonable to expect the public member, on behalf of the community at large, both patients and doctors, to question objectively the delivery of health care services, not as a medical expert but as an informed third party observer. . . . We are taught to accept certain ways of doing things. . . . They should be reviewed and challenged, and public members of regulatory boards of all professions can enhance this evaluation. . . . I believe my responsibility as a public member is to have the social conscience that enables me to balance the interest of both patient and provider. . . . I believe that the ultimate goal of rehabilitation, rather than punishment and revocation, is to be preferred whenever possible. . . . We must be tough and firm and fair. . . . The role and function of the public board member is to be informed, involved and committed. . . . One major concern of self-regulation is the opportunity

for protectionism. . . . Public members are uniquely situated to prevent this scenario, and we must be assertive if the public is to be protected.[29]

Here we have an excellent description of the process through which a public member should consider various public protection options, but he qualifies his public protection stance with making rehabilitation a priority.

The Civic/Public Domain

Most public-interest advocates agree that public members should strive to make boards accountable to the public but disagree on how best to accomplish this goal. Should public members be members of public-interest groups where they learn the discourse and practice of protecting the public and represent a specific constituency? Can they be understood as special kinds of experts who add valuable skills and different perspectives to the mix? If we conceptualize public members and patients as consumers, does it "turn citizens into customers and undermine the sense of obligation and public spirit" of doctors as professionals?[30] Should they style themselves as agents of change, confront the professional members, or just remind them about their broader responsibilities? Not only is who they should be debated, but it is difficult to find public members who can serve many weekdays per year as few employers are willing to permit such service. Some public members took vacation days, and others were retired, had no jobs, owned their own businesses, or held academic positions.

Statutes frequently define public members by what they should not be: "Calling public members a 'great potential resource' for credentialing agencies, the National Commission for Health Certifying Agencies issued in July a set of criteria for public membership on certifying agencies." The list included not being a member of a credentialed profession, not deriving more than 5 percent of income from an agency that dealt with the profession, not having a spouse who was a member of the profession, not being a member of another health profession, not representing that profession for a fee for five years, not working for a firm with substantial interest in the profession, and having previous experience doing board work.[31]

There is a view that as consumers, public members need to be constantly reminded about their distinct perspectives. Esther Peterson, presidential consumer advisor, articulated a difference between consumers and professionals in these terms: "What distinguishes the 'consumer perspective' from an industry or government viewpoint for consumer or citizen representatives serving on regulatory, advisory or planning bodies? The consumer perspective consists of a commitment to fundamental consumer rights and . . . truly representing the view of the user—the consumer."[32] Does this promote a market rather than professional model?

A "constituent" interest-group perspective defines participants as representing either professionals or consumers. During a large meeting concerned with public participation on health boards, some attendees expressed an opinion that public members needed an active constituency to encourage the development and maintenance of a public perspective. Others disagreed, pointing out that such a perspective is a mirror image of self-serving professionals representing narrow interests of their medical societies:

> It is one thing for a professional society to exercise its political muscle from outside a board; it is not, however, acceptable for a professional member of a board to view his or her job as representing the interests of the professional society. . . . If one believes a professional member of a board should take the public perspective, how can one say that public members should sit on the boards as designated representatives of a constituency? The ultimate goal should be to arrive at a day when all board members truly represent the public interest and it does not really matter whether they are members of the profession or lay people.[33]

The need for expertise is another contentious issue that arose at the same meeting. Participants debated what public-member expertise needed to be: listen, learn, lead, communicate with legislators, not be intimidated, attend meetings regularly, or work with media as the most effective tool in educating the public. Others stressed that public representatives' effectiveness depends on their experiences as patients. Just being different could be seen as an asset when it came to a public member's perspective.[34] Being legislators, teachers, lawyers, parents, or patients generally means standing in different places, adopting disparate perspectives, or possessing diverse expertise. Yet Charles Bosk observed surgeons telling residents that in making a judgment call they should ask themselves, "What would you do if the patient were your mother?"[35] The fact that members bring diverse perspectives to board work is an advantage insofar as it ensures problems are examined from multiple perspectives. In this respect deliberations on medical boards are similar to deliberative democracy at large.

Public members often feel different, not fully included in a physician's group. But difference and distance can be resources. One public member explained how his special expertise as a priest brought a new perspective to many issues: "I think they were looking for someone who could offer input from a spiritual perspective on ethical issues. Maybe someone who could make the board members stop and think, 'Are we being fair to this person and to the public?' We refer to it as looking at things with grace."[36] As we can see from this example, bringing different perspectives to board work can be an asset. A woman who served as chair of an investigatory panel described herself to me as an outsider, yet she did not feel excluded. "It was painful on my first panel. It concerned sexual boundary issues by a psychiatrist." Sexual boundary issues are power issues, but if she used the "if it were your daughter" strategy, she told me emphatically, "it would be a cheap shot, and the doctors wouldn't respect me. I'm an outsider, but the doctors respect my opinion. We have healthy dialogues." A case against a woman doctor came up for discussion and, though she had no personal tie with this doctor, she said, "They thought that I would side with her because I'm a woman," but she didn't. She told me she always asked questions, which was not the case with other public members, and kept "the focus on what the problem is and not get lost in extraneous facts and issues. And then it is important to keep your emotions out." A long-term board member emphasized to a group of public members attending a national meeting that public members should use skills from their experiences: "I've found that as I am not a physician, I don't immediately fit . . . [it] can be a great advantage. For example, especially concerning the impaired physician. I myself am not recovering and I thought that this was a disadvantage, and now I think it an advantage. . . . I am not part of the medical establishment. . . . Yesterday I accentuated the fact that I was the only lay candidate [for national office]. . . . I think that it is very good that public members draw attention to their way of life. . . . It is good to individualize ourselves as public members just as the doctors do."

Some public members described their roles as the board's social conscience—their responsibility was advocating for patients. One member pushed the board to justify the disciplinary outcome to the complainant in the required letter. "If you can't justify it to the complainant . . . I want to hear the answers from the physicians. It sort of makes them sit up and sometimes more willing to think that they ought to do something here . . . that is my first question—can you explain it to the complainant?" She was demanding to be persuaded in nonmedical language that the action taken was appropriate to protect the public.

Often public members ask different questions than physicians. One board member explained that when she began on her board, she was afraid of medical cases, asking questions quietly only after the physicians asked theirs. She found she could bring another perspective to the discussion even on medical cases. She explained she sometimes used "would you send your children to . . ." when she became frustrated. Sexual boundary cases became her specialty. "I always feel that you have to be there to protect the women as they are often easy prey—they are victims. The men don't get it. They say, why would a guy like me possibly have sex with a woman like that?"

Public members do not invent the public discursive domain; it is found in public-interest group, government, and Federation publications. This discourse does not exclude the possibility of rehabilitation as much as it shifts the emphasis to protecting the public as the first responsibility. Mark Yessian of the Office of the Inspector General at HHS, writing in the *Federation Bulletin*, distinguishes between the "self-regulation" paradigm that has characterized the professions, and is considered by the professions as part of their identity as professionals, and the "public protection" paradigm, in which "medical licensure authorities are public, not professional, bodies focused on public protection. Whatever the distribution between public and physician board members, the authorities must draw on medical expertise to carry out their responsibilities. But those physicians, who serve, whether as board members, staff or consultants, do so as agents of the public and must be responsive to its concerns."[37]

Slowly board physicians began to insist that all members put public protection first, and some administrators think so, too. Physicians do sometimes use the language of public protection to justify their positions when they decide on licensure and discipline. In a sanction case discussed on Board A, a physician asked the group after a protracted discussion concerning the life of a physician, "Isn't it our job to protect the public? I think this doctor is a danger. I don't care why he did it." The board voted unanimously to revoke. Just two years before, the board was chastised in a newspaper editorial for failing to protect the public, but with more active public members and younger physicians, this board began to shift from the default "understanding" stance to the public protection perspective.

One physician who had come around to the "public protection" frame explained it in terms of what he was seeing on the board. He said that before joining, he would not have believed some of the things that doctors did and that "doctor protectionists" were unaware of what really goes on. In the past, most staff and board members would cringe at what I heard an administrator say to a board member: "We are a law enforcement agency and not in the business of rehabilitation; moreover, even in quality-of-care cases, an issue arises with the difficulty of finding programs for retraining. Additionally, how do you monitor in a rural area? It is often necessary to suspend or revoke to protect the public." Despite socialization into the remediation perspective, doctors can change in the course of board interactions.

Whatever a particular member brings to the board matters, it no longer determines the common reference frame. Each board has a way of looking at cases, a process for assessing cases, and a history of how work gets done. It also has existing social relationships, and new members have to learn about their board and colleagues. Preconceptions of boards and their cases are often swept aside, but on others, they are reaffirmed. A public member put it bluntly:

> You might remind them . . . the three "m's:" medicine, money, and morals. When you are talking about medical matters whether something follows standards of care—beyond that I think that the public members should take their advice, but on the other matters which I think are about two-thirds of the cases . . . they are dealing with fraud or crossing sexual boundaries or alcohol, as you were talking about, and drug addiction. . . . The medical doctors have no special abilities—knowledge to deal with those matters. Matter of fact, I went to a meeting on the impaired physicians program, and they were just fine in the morning because they were dealing with drugs and alcohol. Everyone understood all about that. In the afternoon they started on the sexual boundaries. Immediately one of the doctors raised his hand. 'We don't know much about that. We ought to study that.' So I said, 'If you don't know much about that, you better go over what the rest of us know, because the rest of us know a lot about it.' And in the intermission, the rest of the program the people came over to me and thanked me because they said that they ran into that all over the place. . . . So I don't think that the public members have to defer to anyone or to the medical doctors, unless it concerns medical matters.

A second public member added: "I agree with you, but I would take it one step further. I think that even on the medical issues we have a lot to offer. On the committee they have expert testimony, and the anesthesiologist on the committee may ask more pointed questions, but we all get the same information to digest. I think that all three of the members of the committee can make as educated a decision as the others." This dialogue underscores that many cases do not involve technical knowledge, but expert testimony helps all in cases of incompetence and negligence so that people who are knowledgeable in the ways of the world can understand key issues and ensure the public interest is well expressed.

Sexual Misconduct: Domain Contest

Content of discussion, as well as its form, is at issue in discussing sexual misconduct. In 1994, a Federation committee challenged medicine's cultural authority to define sexual acts between doctors and patients as "medical issues" or as issues between consenting adults, absolving doctors of responsibility. The committee agreed that sex between doctors and patients had to be defined in terms of public protection and was misconduct involving power abuse, not an impairment issue requiring medical treatment. More than fifteen years later, the discourse still occasionally used to decide such cases is that, when patients and physicians are adults and their intimate relations unfold outside the medical office or hospital, they should be immune to professional review, for example, "I know plenty of doctors who married their patients." Physicians sometimes point out that sex with young or multiple patients is an illness and can be treated as a medical problem requiring medical solutions. Similarly, medical frames dominate discourse about drug or alcohol abuse, with abusers seen as having a disease needing treatment.

The Federation Ad Hoc Committee on Physician Impairment, established in 1993, first focused on drug and alcohol issues. In 1994, the FSMB president asked the committee to propose definitions of sexual misconduct and board procedures for dealing with it. The sexual boundary report differentiated between chemical dependency that needed rehabilitation and sexual misconduct that needed discipline: "The committee does not view it as such [an impairment] but instead as a violation of the public trust. It should be noted that although a mental disorder may be a basis for sexual misconduct, the committee finds that sexual misconduct usually is not caused by physical/mental impairment. While sexual addiction is a frequently used phrase, it is not recognized as a disease in the *Diagnostic and Statistical Manual of Psychiatric Disorders, Version IV (DSM IV)*."[38] This definition of sexual misconduct clearly takes the actions away from the disease model: "Sexual misconduct is behavior that exploits the physician-patient relationship in a sexual way. This behavior is nondiagnostic and nontherapeutic, may be verbal or physical, and may include expressions of thoughts and feelings or gestures that are sexual or that reasonably may be construed by a patient as sexual. . . . It is a violation of the public's trust, and causes immeasurable harm, both mentally and physically to the patient."[39]

When the patient's perspective was presented at conferences, someone always asked about how much the patient's interpretation of the physician's act as sexual counts, even if the doctor "didn't mean" it as sexual. That is to say, what matters is the physician's motivation rather than the patient's perception. One state revoked the license of a psychiatrist for having a long-term sexual relationship with a much younger seriously ill female patient, but when the physician moved to another state, the new state permitted him to practice as long as he treated only male patients. A board member in the second state explained that the woman, who was institutionalized in a mental hospital, had sent poems to the doctor after the revocation in the first state. The patient was held partially responsible.

A debate followed an FSMB panel that mentioned medical practice as a "scanning device" for sexual partners. Someone asked, if you removed minors and psychiatric patients, is it such a heinous crime? The discussion focused on the doctor's story until a public member said that patients have the right not to fear doctors and that those found guilty shouldn't be allowed to practice. If a psychiatrist did it once, he will do it again. A female physician declared, "Sex is a violation of trust." This put public interest first. But one administrator told me his board frequently voted to send sexual offenders for rehabilitation, and, when the legislature mandated revocation, he felt relief.

This is not a settled area; the contestation continued when in 2005 the Federation document was reworked by a new committee. Some wanted a more medical view of sexual offenses and to delete references to power. One discussion focused on when patients became "former" patients. The range of sexual misconduct is broad—it can include multiple underage patients, sexual relations with several patients in the office, a sexual relationship with a single adult, sexual touching without intercourse, and sexual language. About half of the actions taken on sexual misconduct cases resulted in minor sanctions.[40] Many boards require supervision or rehabilitation programs; they may not see acts from patients' perspectives.

The Legal/Administrative Discursive Domain and Legal Practices

The number of lawyers, investigators, and administrators working for boards has increased in the last two decades, allowing boards to handle more disciplinary cases and contributing to organizational and language change. Some boards rely on law more than others. Law, particularly due process, is involved in all disciplinary processes, but the more legally oriented the processes, the greater the demands to fit disciplinary talk into legal discursive categories. The more board work shifts to discipline, the greater the role lawyers play as they help interpret statutes and court decisions and organize the disciplinary process.

The balance of staff members who work for boards or the state varies. Board employees are usually evaluated on their knowledge of board procedures and efficiency, but state employees know that their work often is assessed by board ranking and front-page news coverage, and it may be affected by state politics.[41] Staff members who work for boards are subject more to the approval of the board members and medical society politics. Staff members have a different influence over board work; those working for the state often have statutory responsibility for some decisions, while others who work for the boards take on informal responsibility by orchestrating presentations and deciding which cases to investigate fully as the number of reports became too high to leave preliminary decisions to volunteers. Staff members generally do the daily work and follow up on pending cases. One executive told me that he laid out his recommendations in an agenda, which left board members less work to do. In another state where staff authority was informal, an employee concerned about board members wavering after making decisions contacted the media to announce the decision.

Some members express uneasiness about the increasing influence and authority of staff. A former chief regulatory officer believed that authority for decisions relating to occupational regulation should rest with "the commissioner of the state licensing agency." Professional groups would advise at each stage, but "the real issue is that the state regulatory board should not be the final authority.'"[42] Once a board was no longer independent from the state, the question was who should have what authority: the board, the state agency, or staff? What kinds of decisions should and does staff make during daily routines? "Attorneys and other career civil servants handle the machinery of board operations, including the collection of allegations, the review of their validity, investigations when staff find them warranted, conferences with alleged transgressors, and, if no agreement is reached, administrative hearings."[43] The authors of this statement bemoaned board members' lack of involvement.

Public members sounded their concerns about staff authority to prioritize cases and remove "too many cases" from consideration. With staff involvement in the disciplinary process, the outcome increasingly hinges on the administrators' pronouncements—"boards received more complaints than can be fully investigated," "long hearings are expensive," or "a settlement eliminates an expensive court appeal." Efficiency in using available resources is often cited by administrators as the reason for eliminating or taking up particular cases.

Investigators with various skills are crucial in case construction; investigating fraud or sexual misconduct requires different skills than those needed for negligence or incompetence cases. On some boards, investigators actively participate in discussions of the cases with board members, while others only collect evidence. One administrator explained to me that he had no medical advisor and could do no medical cases. "So much is swept under the rug. We are looked at by physicians as police, and all the docs are tied into networks so that few cases [of negligence or incompetence] are ever done."

Some cases are pursued because they are easier to dispose of, which makes the board's productivity look respectable. Quality-of-care cases (negligence and incompetence) are the most difficult and expensive to prosecute; they require expensive expert witnesses and extensive investigations, so some are turned into "poor record keeping," which is easier to document and prosecute. But the sanction may be weaker. Boards sometimes prosecute easy cases such as "diet doctor" cases—doctors who provide prescriptions without proper documentation to people who never lose weight. Such cases are rarely controversial as many physicians do not greatly respect such doctors. A prosecutor may judge a lesser sanction preferable when, because of the statutes, a fixed suspension of two years means the doctor cannot ask for his license back for two years, and, if it is revoked, he can return in six months to ask for it back, which requires a costly hearing. Efficiency talk often carries the day.

The extent to which legal discourse and practice penetrate board decision making differs. A handful of states structure both investigatory committees and hearings by the strictures of law. Most states use mixed procedures, with the investigatory stage structured more as "peer review" and the hearings driven more by legal discourse. When legal procedures are the main reference frame, board members are told that their job is to help construe the facts and decide whether the allegations have been proved by the civil standards of "preponderance of the evidence" or "clear and convincing." Training sessions bear on how to write an opinion, to decide a sanction, conduct a hearing, and make a legal argument. The emphasis is on what happened, if the facts can be proved, and if the record is clear. Evaluating credibility of witnesses is important. At a dispositional hearing in front of the entire board after a panel had made a finding of a violation of the medical practice act, a physician talked about the doctor's behavior, which he observed in the hospital. Since this information was not on the record, the board member was stopped by a lawyer. Legal discourse is not something learned in medical training, nor do physicians have much experience with formal sanctions. Legal discourse and practice must be taught.

Some board physicians want to dispense with legal procedures: "Take away his license—he's a bad doc." When they see no excuse for an action, they are apt to waive the legal framework altogether. Astounded by a case making national news that exposed a physician who left a patient on the operating table while he left to cash a check, board members wanted to revoke immediately.[44] The lack of concern with legal processes sometimes leads to discussions as to why a panel hearing a case needs to establish the credibility of witnesses in their written opinion.

The domains of medicine, public protection, and law are often in competition. Tensions develop among members and between members and staff in the use of particular frames for interpretation and action. The dominant domain of each board varies and not only serves as explanation for action but contributes to the construction of what they do and how, the range of possibilities, and what is emphasized. Domains also inform us about what should happen, how particular cases need to be constructed, how they move through the system, and what the decision-making process involves. It does not mean that everyone on a board uses the same framework or that they stay on the same page. Participants move back and forth, and often doctors and administrators revert to familiar turf.

Confronting Board Work

Whatever the area of expertise and preferred form of talk, board members all face new issues, procedures, regulations, laws, and a range of disciplinary cases. During work and informal conversations, members learn who the others are and how they talk. Some medical members, surprised by the cases they see, readily accept the public protection discourse. Public members vacillate between accepting medical talk and using their skills to advocate for public protection. The president of FSMB in 1999, Dr. Alan Schumacher, maintained that physicians are unprepared for board work when he discussed the case of Dr. Swango, who was found guilty in court of murdering patients: "Because physicians instinctively seem to exhibit an almost naive reluctance to believe ill of a colleague . . . the fear of being sued and the fear of reflecting badly on oneself . . . leads to this ongoing failure in professional self-regulation—the failure of peer review as a system of public protection."[45]

While doctors fall back on what they know, some are surprised by the failures of doctors who appear before the board.[46] Membership may become a wake-up call to better protect the public, as cases are substantially different from typical hospital peer reviews or M&M conferences. I watched one doctor working as an expert reviewing a case gasp when he heard the details. Afterward he asked if this were the type of case generally handled and, when told it was, he said he would not have believed doctors did those things. A physician with twenty years of practice, who served on quality assurance committees, was astonished by his first case—a doctor stalking his wife. "This is an egregious case," he exclaimed. Later he told me that most doctors work so hard, it is particularly terrible when they do things like this. Another said that he was similarly situated to a doctor under investigation and that the doctor should not have been doing pain management because he was a drug abuser. "I stand without doubt that he should not be practicing—he is a sociopath." "The medical board is not for the thin skinned," a doctor told me, and a retired physician added, "I would have been a better doctor if I had been on the board earlier." A solo practitioner who did not know any board members before joining often found the board work overwhelming. He said at first that he did not want to say anything because he might ask something embarrassing and remained reluctant to speak out. Like the others, he was surprised by doctors' lying to patients about their illnesses, the drug and alcohol problems, and operations, for example, on the "wrong leg." He thought the board was not sufficiently tough on sexual offenders after he heard what a former FSMB president said about the failure to rehabilitate sexual offenders. Board members are taken aback by the incivility of doctors. One board wanted to sanction doctors who spoke crudely to staff, reducing several to tears. The shock of what doctors have done who appear before the boards makes enough of an impression to differentiate board work from other medical evaluation experiences. But few talked of patients' suffering.

Lack of familiarity with many issues exacerbates the public members need for training in public protection. A board administrator explained to me: "Public members are awed at first; I keep drawing them out. They have greater sense sometimes and express their concerns. They also ask good questions. Sometimes they 'get a feeling,' but we are doing less training. They slowly develop a progressive sense of value and importance. We have to encourage public members to participate and keep participating. The lack of training is a real problem."

While physicians have several members to serve as models, many boards have only one or two public members, so new members have little opportunity to see if public members ask different types of questions. Some public members have a difficult time envisioning what they can add, but others can find their skills useful. Public members have helped develop the operations of the board. Among the more frequently mentioned items at a CAC meeting were rewriting the letters that patients received about their cases, ensuring that all reports from citizens were acknowledged, prioritizing the complaints from the consumers' perspective, instituting Robert's rules of order at meetings, establishing due process on the board, opening the board to public scrutiny, and writing and stewarding new legislation through the legislature. The reasoning skills necessary for questioning doctors are essential to board work. One woman described how to bring the patient's perspective into the discussions: "It is called the 'X standard.' In the discussions, if I feel that I don't want the doctor treating my family, my friends, or neighbors, [then] it doesn't meet the X standard." Unprompted, the executive of her board mentioned to me later that day that the "X standard" worked well.

Several public members with political connections used their clout to enhance board resources and aid board activities. A member serving on a chronically underfunded board pushed the legislature to raise annual licensing fees and helped the board organize as a modern board staffed with professionalized administrators and was elected president. A woman who had worked for her governor explained that she uses her legislative skills: "We have had a number of confidentiality issues recently and we tracked over two hundred bills—actively ten or twelve. It opens a Pandora's Box. . . . It was mind boggling that the issue was labeled confidentiality. Yet, I think I want to say seventy bills were introduced that I followed—that is one of the ways that a public member can contribute."

I heard stories similar to my own when as a member I was pushed by the board to confront the medical society. One of the most important issues that divided Board A and the state medical society was the Advanced Nurse Practice Act, which gave nurses with advanced degrees the right to open an independent practice and prescribe some medications with a physician collaborative agreement. The medical society took a public stand against the act. I was urged to speak to the legislative committee in favor of the act that the board had worked on with the nurses when a member of the medical society claimed all doctors were against independent practice. The bill passed.

The Public Discursive Domain Endures

The extent to which the various discursive domains enter board work and how they affect interactions varies, but no board can bypass the deliberative process. The interest-group voting model has limited value for understanding board activities, for it ignores the role of making sense together. Board members sometimes change their minds when asked to think differently. A foreign-trained physician came before the entire board requesting an exemption because he was one point short on one section of his national exam but was already licensed in two states. He had invented a surgical technique and was published in excellent medical journals. The board had never granted an exemption, except to practice in "underserved areas." This articulate doctor was trained in a country with excellent medical schools. After much discussion, the board physicians were clearly inclined to say no, as they had in the first licensing case I saw. The deputy attorney general insisted that state statutes did not provide for an exemption in this case. By this point I had more confidence and asked if the board doctors would like this doctor in our state if a family member needed this surgery. The answer was yes. We were warned if we granted him a license, it could be challenged in court. Here we can see the distinction between law and public interest. As board members we could settle for a safe "no." As citizens, thinking about the common interest, we wanted to grant the license. We changed the rule soon afterwards.

Decisions usually come after deliberation, and the quality of the deliberative process matters; we need to know who takes an active part in deliberations and who lays back, which questions are raised and which are not, what counts as evidence, and which arguments sway the group. How closely do board deliberations approximate deliberative democracy at large? Discussions about deliberative democracy often ignore the importance of group members' experiences and ways of talking and constructing presentations developed outside the deliberating group. When people join new groups, they do not drop their habits—their acquired knowledge, skills, ways of talking, demeanors, and self-presentation routines.

Can public members formulate questions and arguments and assess cases and issues from the perspective of multiple publics? Do public members merely lend legitimacy to a process controlled by the profession, or do they make a substantive contribution? A long-term staff member explained to me that, over the years, public members increasingly took independent stances and physicians used to be more patronizing of public members, but he also expressed a contradictory observation. Public members are brought into the club, and the board has become a cohesive unit—is this co-optation or cooperation? Public and medical members may adopt a "protect the public" stance, but some board organizations actively promote this reference frame, while others make it difficult for its public members to make their voices heard. Are there types of boards where all are more likely to think broadly as citizens?

Chapter 6

Medical and Legal Discourses in Investigatory Committees

By the end of the twentieth century board members took their disciplinary authority seriously, framing their goal as public protection. About 12 percent of cases largely concerned incompetence and negligence, but the majority focused on what Dr. Edmund Pellegrino considered character issues or what Charles Bosk characterized as failures of moral performance.[1] According to Pellegrino, "Board members must repress the temptation to protect the profession or retaliate for sometimes vindictive attacks on professional integrity by the media, patient groups, or other professions. . . . Failures of character are more numerous, more subtle, and perhaps, in sum total more damaging to the public interest than incompetence. . . . The central place of character in the professional relationship poses a dilemma for conscientious licensing boards. . . . These assessments are crucial in decisions about degrees of guilt, and severity of discipline."[2] George Bernard Shaw's satire is different;

> *B.B.*: Have you forgotten the lovely opera singer I sent you to have that growth taken off her vocal cords?
>
> *Walpole*: Great heavens, man, you don't mean to say you sent her for a throat operation!
>
> *B.B.*: . . . You removed her nuciform sac. . . . She got back her voice after it, and thinks you are the greatest surgeon alive.[3]

The "nuciform sac" may be fictional, but cases of wrong-sited surgery and misdiagnosis are not infrequent.[4] How public members are to assess negligence and incompetence raises issues, as does how "character" is established.

Misconduct categories vary, with some states providing only general classes of actionable misconduct and others spelling out offenses in detail. The boards with which I had firsthand experience had ranges from fewer than fifteen designated categories of misconduct to more than fifty.[5] The procedures for handling such cases differed as well across the country. "We don't do it that way," a board member might claim, or an administrator might chime in, "Our statute doesn't allow such infractions as grounds for discipline."

Ordinarily, boards have four-stage disciplinary processes, although the stages are not always sharply separated, who acts at each stage varies, and what the participants can do also varies. At the first stage, the task is to determine which "reports" should be fully investigated. Staff often manages this stage. Having determined that a report has some merit, an administrator gives it to investigators to collect evidence. Who then decides whether to bring a case to a board's attention varies. At the second stage, an investigatory panel or committee, often composed of two physicians and one public member—but there are many variations—examines the evidence and, sometimes, interviews the doctor. Some boards use outside experts at this stage, while many rely more on staff physicians or board members' expertise to evaluate negligence and incompetence. An investigatory panel's recommendation is not easy to predict. This chapter focuses on these two stages of the disciplinary review process. They are critical, as most cases end during the second stage with a dismissal, a confidential reprimand, or a public settlement.[6] From talking to participants over many years, I have discerned that case presentations fit a number of patterns, and I have developed examples based on board members' and staff's accounts. These examples illustrate the types of discussions and problems facing deliberants on medical boards, particularly public members. The types of problems that the doctors under investigation face that I use here are common ones seen by boards.

The third stage is the hearing, which can take place before the entire board (this was true of Board C), a hearing committee (this was true of Boards A, B, and D), or a legally trained hearing officer. Most cases are settled prior to a hearing. The findings of fact or conclusions of law from a hearing can be overturned by the full board in some states. The fourth stage entails the disciplinary decision. In many states the disciplinary decision is made by the entire board after a committee hears the case and makes recommendations (this was true for Boards A and D). In other states, the same people who hear the case make disciplinary decisions (this was true for Boards B and C).

At each stage in the process board members engage in deliberation. The deliberative democracy model accentuates equality among the members of the deliberative body and envisions participants who are immune to emotional distortions and resist strategic, self-interested outcomes. The deliberation, according to this model, must be rational and conflict free. That is not always what I observed and learned from presentations and comments at national meetings. In real-life settings, participants are not necessarily equal and some-times let their emotions flare, pushed self-interested agendas, and failed to join issue with each other.[7] Not surprisingly, public interest can get lost in such proceedings. The public-interest frame tends to be weaker than the medical and legal frames, less articulated, and not as logically consistent, with members having a difficult time figuring out where to insert community-based arguments, even though some boards fare better than others in making room for public-interest arguments.[8] Aside from sexual misconduct cases, victims who are stirred by strong emotions and who could focus board's attention on public protection rarely have a chance to appear before boards.[9]

Medical and legal arguments shape the disciplinary process differently. Medical discourse often relies on board members as experts, all sides of the issue do not necessarily receive equal attention as the attention is focused on the physician, and public members feel discouraged airing their concerns in the midst of medically driven discourse. The language is that of "understand-ing and rehabilitation." With legal-administrative discourse, the power shifts to administrators and board attorneys whose prime agenda is efficiency and legal soundness. The focus is on evidence. Medically trained administrators and investigators tend to think differently once they are schooled in this kind of discourse, seeing things from the legal/administrative standpoint.[10] While each discourse may obscure issues central to public members, the legal domain offers richer resources to public members and affords broader opportunities for articulating the public protection agenda. It is also a potent tool for protecting physicians from being railroaded.

Dealing with Reports

Complaints about a doctor's performance come from differing sources: patients and their families, doctors and other health-care workers, hospitals and insur-ance companies, the courts, and other states. Depending on the state, reports may be verbal, written, filed over the Internet, or anonymous. In the first three quarters of the twentieth century, board members often dealt with all the reports that came their way, read every letter, and then set out to investigate. That is the practice I encountered when I joined Board A. By the 1980s, most states received more reports than members could handle, and it increasingly fell to staff to evaluate which cases might involve a violation of the medical practice act and, thus, merited further investigation. Even if valid, many reported infractions do not violate the local medical practice act. For instance, in some states overcharging was not a valid ground for misconduct; hence, cases of this kind were dismissed with a brief note to the petitioner.[11] A physician with poor communication skills might receive a confidential letter or be invited for an interview in some states, but most of these reports probably resulted in dismissal. According to the *Federation Bulletin*, staff in one state developed a "two-call" approach for serious communication issues and misunderstandings— a physician staff member called both the physician and the patient to see if the matter could be resolved without further board involvement.[12]

As the number of reports grew and workloads swelled, the number of staff supporting board work expanded, and efficiency became a powerful discourse and practice. Staff backgrounds were diverse—medical, administrative, legal, or law enforcement. To increase efficiency, many boards developed triage systems in the 1990s to investigate the most serious cases quickly. States with limited resources had to rely on board members and share investigators with other agencies to collect and interpret evidence. Staff sometimes decides which cases to bring before a board committee and often presents cases, summarizes investigations, and furnishes documents upon which the panel relies.

Investigations vary in the information provided to boards. When I joined Board A, we read every report, and the entire board decided what to do about a particular case and who among us would investigate. The process changed when we hired a director who, along with a board member, determined whether to investigate the case and then did the investigation. From that point on, little evidence was presented to the board when we decided whether to call for a hearing. We went from knowing everything about incoming reports to having little information. The board had to trust the director. On Board B, staff made decisions about cases meriting investigation and assigned cases to investigators, trained in the area in which they investigated. In the case of Boards C and D, staff made initial decisions, but an investigatory committee of board members stayed involved and often interviewed problem doctors as part of the investigation process, thus merging investigation with the investigatory panel (the second stage). This was the case in many states.

Although many reported cases are dismissed, other cases of possible misconduct go unreported. Doctors, hospitals, and other health-care professionals are reluctant to report problem physicians, making it possible for those physicians to continue practicing. "It was years before he was stopped," writes Atul Gawande about an orthopedic surgeon who was protected over many years by his colleagues while patients were harmed.[13]

Medical Discursive Domain

In most instances cases are dismissed, a settlement is reached, or an informal reprimand is given by an Investigative Committees (IC).[14] Investigative committees on Boards A, C, and D often used medical/professional discourse to frame cases, as did many other boards. These ICs seemed to have fewer debates about legal issues, such as sufficiency of evidence. Board or staff members were often pressed into service as experts to evaluate possible negligence and incompetence cases, and they only sometimes discussed the standard of care fully at meetings. A medical staff member presents the case, a fairly common procedure among the states. I use "medical director" or "medical coordinator" to illustrate this role, but sometimes board members present. The presentation of "rounds" was a standard format for structuring the presentation to the investigatory panel, as I learned from discussions with board members across the country. Like everyone else, doctors tend to fall back on familiar formats and language.[15] Sometimes the problem physician was called in for an interview, which at times doubled as a monitoring exercise with the problem physician urged to enter a rehabilitation program or attend additional training, or the physician was simply served with a private letter of concern.[16] Like a mortality and morbidity (M&M) conference, the investigative panel strove to "understand" what happened, and members drew on their experiences to imagine what must have happened. If no one could come up with an explanation, the doctor was invited to show that nothing happened out of the ordinary, and, failing that, IC members wanted to "see" that the doctor understood what he had done wrong.

In such proceedings, lawyers are not always present, and physicians may have only vague notions about legal standards and administrative procedures. In certain classes of cases (e.g., drug sales), board members often wanted to move directly to discipline and revoke the license, dispensing with due process. They tended to trust their own judgment more than evidentiary hearings, and often decried legal niceties and procedural rules as superfluous. In one case, a doctor told me he pressed for a hearing to discipline a physician for fraud, but the investigators had insufficient evidence to do so. The case did not go to a hearing, but the member voiced his suspicions. This case required no medical knowledge, and the public member had successfully used legal discourse, warning board members about hasty decisions based on little evidence. Legal considerations prevented the case from going forward.

The IC process can take the form of informal "eye-to-eye" encounters with problematic doctors, who may be led to understand that they will be forgiven if they admit their mistakes. Some board members developed routine questions, which others learned and imitated. One public member said she always queried physicians under review about their home life; a medical director told me that incompetency or negligence cases typically resulted in informal agreements to seek additional training or therapy. "We are a rehabilitative board," explained a staff member. With few legal barriers, this process allowed for the addition of what members knew from the community or the understanding of what "typically happens" to aid in the interpretation of events. With this scripted story, as Dr. Pellegrino notes, members can discuss the character of the physician, a subject about which physicians have little particular expertise and about which public members can take a stand but often have little information to use to do so.

The Doctor's Tale

Doctors learn to tell stories about patients in the course of their training. The IC presentation structure encourages this habit. The tale that is told, like the patient's story developed for rounds, is that of a presenter and the doctor under investigation. Often elegant and well rehearsed, such stories contain several recurrent themes. The story starts with a brief statement about the nature of the problem the doctor faced—for example, substance abuse, drug sales, sexual misconduct, fraud, incompetence, or negligence. Next, the panel hears at length about the history of the physician's career, after which the presenter briefly sums up the specific issue raised by the complainant and, drawing on his experience, offers a diagnostic conclusion about the outlined symptoms. The format follows the pattern of hospital rounds, which favor the biographical and historical. "It may yield a useful explication of otherwise obscure details that cannot be long ignored, like marital stress, loss of work, a child's illness." The story proceeds in chronological order from the immediate past to the history and then the tests and, in the case of misconduct, to the outcome. If a fact does not fit, the reviewer develops a hypothesis to explain it away, just as happens during rounds.[17] If presenters can develop a sensible account or excuse for something that took place, be this misconduct or medical error, the case stops right there. Should members need further information to strengthen or test the account, boards may choose to interview the doctor. The interview process often yields another sensible reason for the mishap that will render harmless or understandable the adverse outcome. Along the way the board comes to believe that the doctor understands what went wrong. I heard accounts like this repeatedly.

Listening to the storyteller, one might conclude the doctor under investigation had an unblemished career until he arrived at a point in his life where he encountered a personal problem, faced some hardship that tripped him, or just happened to be the victim of circumstances beyond his control. "It wasn't really a big event," we might be told, but "something went wrong." One doctor had an exemplary career, was always on top of the situation, but missed a malignancy which was easy to miss. If no one questions the presentation, the panel moves to dismiss. With no outside expert, the panel could take the summary of the event in question as an accurate reconstruction.

A single story with a long presentation of a physician's biography centers the discussion on physician character and allows the patient to fade into the background. In "he said, she said" cases, the account leaves ample room for the character of the doctor to emerge, with little information about the sometimes uninterviewed patient. A medical director may start his presentation with recounting the flaws in the woman patient's character—the allegation that some years back this patient accused another doctor of sexual harassment. A few years later she came to see the second doctor with a medical complaint. The doctor queried the patient about her sexual activities. The woman said in her letter that asking about her sexual history was harassment. Then the medical coordinator might go on to elaborate the doctor's history: He has been in practice for many years. In our records there are no other reports and he has good records. There is no support for her allegation. The case ends without further discussion; no one asks for additional evidence or insists on interviewing the patient. The decision turns on the doctor's alleged good character and her alleged character flaws.

With the focus on the physician, the appeal to character is a strong argument that can outweigh evidence of poor medical skills. A comparison of two cases of new doctors who arguably do not meet the requirements for licensure illustrates the importance of assumptions about character and reliance on intuition and experience to establish doctors' credentials. In the first case, the presenter may portray the doctor as a drinker seeking a license to make money. Members have reservations about his character and vote against granting him a license. A second illustration reveals a doctor with repeated United States Medical Licensing Examination (USMLE) failures and questionable work skills.[18] Still, he was judged to be person of good character. Assessment of character was a common theme in many stories I heard:

> *Medical Director*: We have a reservation about this doctor. He failed the USMLE on more than one occasion. In fact he failed two parts. We saw that he was self-possessed and has good recommendations by his residency program including a superior. He was not recognized as a problem.

Physician Member 1: Depending on how you count his failures, it could be counted as eight times. Do we need to do something?

Physician Member 1: I would rely more on clinical skills and evaluations than a test.

Medical Director: The head of the residency-training program says he is OK.

Physician Member 2: What is the impression that he gives to the public?

Public Member 1: He seems sincere and wants to help people.

Physician Member 1: I agree. There is a world of difference between the two. Here we have a stupid but sincere man with honesty and integrity and I would send a relative to him. The first is not of good character.

Physician Member 2: If he got in over his head would he refer?

Public Member 1: You would send a relative, but he's stupid?

Physician Member 2: It's an intuitive feeling. He's not bright, and there is a poverty of intellect, and there is an obligation to protect the public and to the law, and we can't subvert the law.

Physician Member 1: When did he complete part 1 of the USMLE?

Lawyer: There is no national consensus on how many times a person should take an exam and within what period.

Medical Director: It's always been loose and the Federation doesn't have a position.

Physician Member 2: I move to give him a license.

With reservations, they may approve his license. Though the applicant failed the exam many times before he passed, he seemed to possess good character and recommendations, thus deserving a license. The doctor willing to send his relative to the applicant-doctor takes a patient's perspective. Note that challenging the board member risks impugning his judgment. In the absence of relevant information, a personalized judgment by a physician effectively closes off the opportunity for debate. The public member has little information with which to contest the decision.

While negligence and incompetency cases may hinge on the doctor's character, cases involving sexual misconduct are sometimes decided on the strength of doctor's skills and qualifications. With only a brief summary of the reported incident and no interview of the patient, the presenter has the power to sway the board by focusing on the problem doctor's superior education and professional skills or almost flawless character. By the time the sexual misconduct allegations come into view, the board has already formed a positive opinion about the doctor. When this happens, public members say they have a harder time moving the discussion back to the allegations of sexual misconduct.

A medical director might start with a long story about the superior medical competence of the physician, after which he takes a breath and might add—but he had a very complicated relationship with women. The doctor used sexual innuendos and had been sent to therapy for rehabilitation—a private, nonreportable solution. He accepted that his behavior toward women was inappropriate, but he did it again, the panel is told. One of the board physicians might add, "I can't help but worry, but it wasn't substandard care," accepting the redefinition as a medical case. Another says, "I don't think that there is anything that we can do. He is a superb doctor and he was reported by nurses. He is working in another state, but can't we tell them anything?" A lawyer would inform them they cannot, for the diversion was informal and that nothing was done officially. The medical director then backs off the "good physician" argument, emphasizing instead that the board has no evidence. Since the physician was not sanctioned the first time, there was nothing on his record, a legal response. The patients' perspectives get short shrift, but no one has specific evidence. It was often difficult to find someone to testify. Here a physician, who may have violated doctor-patient trust, escapes further investigation after the discussion confirms his superior medical skills, and they do not have much evidence anyway. Convincing victims to testify requires tenacity, and without their testimony, the legal process cannot go forward. Boards sometimes do not have investigators trained to investigate sexual misconduct cases, and general physician character and skills may be used to decide to dismiss the case.

Another problem hobbling public members is the brevity and speed with which cases are summarized. Consider the following story involving a son and a mother who objected to his treatment and demanded an alternative. The treating doctor dismissed him as a patient, appropriately, according to the case presenter. No one questioned what treatment was given, what was desired by the mother, or what the behavior was that the mother categorized as "abandonment." The presenter's definition and evaluation were accepted. An independent assessment would have required board members to ask probing questions of the presenter's summary and, perhaps, more investigation.

When a medical care issue brings a doctor to the board's attention, the public member often has little information with which to challenge a summary assessment of the presenter. The physician members are better equipped, but their commitment to a fellow professional may override concern for discussing public good or questioning a colleague's assessment. But in some cases they can and may do so. When physicians challenge the presenter's assessment of good character with questions about what the physician under investigation had done, the public members often find it difficult to contribute, as they have no expertise to assess the medical issue. A physician with an impeccable history may do something that the committee cannot explain away readily:

> *Medical Coordinator*: I do believe he is a competent physician. Surgery was warranted, and it was an unfortunate outcome. The patient suffered and got a settlement from the insurance company. Do we have enough evidence or do we need an expert?
>
> *Physician Member 2*: It seemed as though it was an unfortunate outcome then I thought . . .
>
> *Medical Coordinator*: We know in the past that he was good.
>
> *Physician Member 1*: He probably shouldn't have used. . . .
>
> *Medical Coordinator*: No question. An expert could tell you since you asked. He has a fine reputation. Give me a sense of your comfort level.
>
> *Physician Member 2*: There is no sense of carelessness.
>
> *Physician Member 1*: I have an inclination to say no unprofessional conduct, but I would feel better with an outside evaluation. The patient is forty. Why would she stop breathing?
>
> *Physician Member 2*: I would feel better with a consult.

With the explanation of the outcome in doubt, a doctor asked for an expert. When a question about what happened yields no answer, the appeal to character fails. A public member has difficulty raising such questions because the issue involves the need for medical knowledge to do so effectively. Doctors do challenge others when they have knowledge or information that does not fit with the summary presentation.

Adding What Is Typical

When facts are hard to come by, panel members may fill in the blanks with statements of what "typically happens" under similar circumstances, and this opens the door to "reasonable" excuses based on the board members' personal experiences, particularly without a lawyer present. The doctors often volunteered examples from their own medical experiences and used what "typically happens" to fill in their understanding in the absence of evidence. This made it difficult for public members to participate in the discussion, ask for evidence, or provide an alternative interpretation, but they can focus the discussion on the problem. A daughter complained about a physician treating her father. Her father had fallen, and the doctor failed to conduct a careful analysis of his symptoms: he did not fully examine his hip and, two days later, another doctor found fractures. The first doctor's notes were not good, according to the medical director presenting the case:

Physician Member 2: The range of motion was good, according to the notes.

Medical Director: He is probably a little old man who doesn't like to complain. There were lots of problems of miscommunication, and the second doctor turns out to be the hero. He needed surgery.

Public Member 1: What about the initial evaluation? It is the problem today?

Medical Director: The leg and hip were not sufficiently tested, and the report didn't say that he had the full range of motion. X-rays should have been done.

Public Member 1: I'm surprised he signed the discharge.

Medical Director: They must have moved the leg, but not enough to see that the hip was broken. He must have exclaimed if they stopped. Maybe they thought it was bruised.

Public Member 1: A confidential letter.

Physician Member 1: I don't go along.

Public Member 1: If he said it hurt, that should be an indication that he should have done an X-ray.

Physician Member 1: He probably thought it was a bruise.

The medical director may offer an "understanding" of the situation by filling in with typical experiences like "they must have moved the leg" and "thought it was a bruise." The public member uses common sense to introduce the patient's perspective and inquire about the evidence, but doesn't say, "Let's interview the patient to see if your hypothesis holds." Without evidence, the public member is unable to provide an alternative construction. Public members said that at times that they felt that investigations did not provide them with enough evidence to challenge interpretations that did not appear to be directly based on the evidence.

The Interview as Education for the Doctor and Character Assessment by the Board

An interview with a physician is often called for when board members cannot come up with reasonable excuses for the behavior of physicians under investigation or to assure themselves that doctors understand their errors. This further encourages assessment of a case based on the panels' evaluations of doctors' "understandings" or rationales for what they did as in M&M conferences, rather than focusing on exploring what happened from multiple sides. It encourages either sympathy for physicians who "understand" what they did or lack of sympathy when their characters are viewed as questionable according to many board members. When respondents communicated understanding by providing good excuses for what went on or appeared sympathetic (chastened by the experience), board members tended to look at the situation from the physicians' perspectives. Sometimes both board members and staff described the interview process as determinative of the outcome: "If they admit and repent, they survive." They could, in some states, be sent to retraining or rehabilitation programs without a reportable disciplinary action or given a minor sanction.

Even in cases that do not involve medical knowledge and where public members can ask questions, form opinions, and argue, the focus often remains on a physician's character. Incidents of sexual misconduct, fraud, and continual drug abuse or poor prescribing practices arise often. A physician who accepted a consent order after self-prescribing narcotics over a long period attended a rehabilitation clinic and wanted his license back; he wanted to return to work, but no one would hire him as the clinic where he had gone for treatment said that he was not rehabilitated. Despite the established "facts," during the interview, one physician member had to be persuaded that revocation was warranted:

> *Physician Member 1*: I doubt he should get his license back.
> *Board Lawyer*: We stopped counting the number of prescriptions he wrote for himself.
> *Physician Member 1*: He knew what he was doing.
> *Medical Director*: He denied it and did it again that day.

During the interview the doctor requested a limited license in radiology, which would have involved little patient contact or need for writing prescriptions:

> *Board Lawyer*: There were other changes that demonstrate a lack of candor in addition.
> *Public Member 1*: I found it interesting that the only reason he wants his license back is that he owes money . . . I don't see any rehabilitation.
> *Physician Member 2*: Why can't he just do radiology? He won't see patients.
> *Medical Director*: He has either forfeited the right to practice or, when we grant a license, he is entitled to practice. A license limited to radiology doesn't really exist.

Public Member 1: We were considering a limit to when he could come before the board again for a license. Do we want that in the order?

Board Lawyer: He needs a decision.

Public Member 1: I move to deny a license.

Physician Member 2: I think that he could function in society, so radiology is OK with me.

Medical Director: He should go to areas other than medicine.

Public Member 1: Absolutely, medicine shouldn't be polluted.

Physician Member 2: What about research?

Public Member 1: I would be scared about access to drugs.

Board Lawyer: I've asked around, and with his background, no one connected with medicine will hire him.

Medical Director: We were too gentle during the interview.

Physician Member 2: He lied to me and looked me in the eye.

Public Member 1: He is not an honorable man to have an MD after his name. He doesn't have a shred of integrity.

Faced with a doctor, board physicians often wanted to do something for him or her. Not granting a license was an emotional experience, and it was common that groups continued to discuss a case after a vote. Suggesting a revocation or refusing to return a license was not routine, and board members, when faced with the doctor, felt sympathy. Here the issue was character. Public members sometimes expressed their positions from the vantage point of the profession and did not argue that the doctor was a danger to patients. The result protects the public, but the argument was from the profession's perspective.

The informal interview can be a powerful tool for assessing character. When the doctor makes a good impression at the informal interview, the tendency is to evaluate more in terms of character than in terms of what happened or the potential consequences for patients. Sometimes a committee may not have an explanation for why a good doctor would sell medications over the Internet, thus violating the standard of examining patients before prescribing. Prescribing over the Internet without seeing patients has been a problem in many states. A medical coordinator may describe the critical report by a Federation committee on telemedicine and critique articles that a doctor claimed justified Internet prescribing. While he appears to be leaning toward a serious sanction, after an interview, he tells the committee that the doctor believed that Internet prescribing provided an important service:

Medical Coordinator: He made some pleasant comments. He has rules against prescribing controlled substances, and he says he does assess patients. There is no face-to-face exam. It is his way to make money in retirement. He says he prescribes Viagra and a few other drugs. I don't like it.

After the interview, in which the panel established that he had no face-to-face contact with patients, that he was making a lot of money, that the drugs he mostly prescribed did not have significant side effects, and that he was willing to stop his Internet prescribing, the committee appears much less concerned about his actions:

> *Medical Coordinator*: He sounds like a pretty good doctor.
>
> *Lawyer*: Fee splitting with the company is illegal. We could define this as a medical case and not actually seeing the patient or as business case based on the fee splitting.
>
> *Medical Coordinator*: I cannot accept what he does.

A possible recommendation in line with a benign impression might be a reprimand with probation. This reportable sanction was justifiable, I was told by some board members, with doctors that seemed cooperative and expressed understanding of doing wrong. The problem doctor's understanding and contrition were sometimes judged as the guarantee the reprimand would be a sufficient deterrent.

If the doctor does not acknowledge his responsibility, the doctors on the board are apt to infer he doesn't "understand" the significance of his actions. There have been numerous cases of equipment salesmen in operating rooms and questions about what they are doing there. A physician used new equipment without testing it in advance and blamed the salesman in the room during his interview with the panel. However, the salesman did nothing during surgery. The device, the panel discovered, was complicated, and they viewed the older device as adequate. It was the doctor's responsibility to practice before deciding whether to use it:

> *Physician Member 1*: He tried to say, "The hospital didn't stop me."
>
> *Medical Coordinator*: It would have been different if it had been his fifteenth accident.
>
> *Physician Member 2*: It is unprofessional to use it without experimenting. It was a totally different type of instrument.
>
> *Medical Coordinator*: Other doctors objected to its use.
>
> *Board Lawyer*: We have an outside consultant report that says he chose to use it without practicing.
>
> *Medical Coordinator*: The doctor is the final protector of the patient.

Physician Member 2: He didn't hold it in his hands before surgery. . . . I
    move that we affirm unprofessional conduct.

Physician Member 1: I guess, I agree.

Public Member 1: The patient suffered.

[The medical coordinator explains the difference in instruments again.]

Physician Member 2: I'm very concerned with his conduct—using
    an instrument without testing it in advance. That shows very poor
    judgment.

The doctor was evaluated as failing to understand the seriousness of his
actions, unlike the prior doctor. Board members often told me a doctor's
failure to acknowledge responsibility when things under his control went
wrong was a sign that they needed to take action and suggest a hearing if they
could not settle the case. The board doctors show concern from the patients'
perspectives when confronted by actions that they assess as inexcusable and
when the physician fails to take responsibility. Public members are able,
despite the focus on the physician, to insert the patient's perspective.

Challenging or Accepting Expertise

Board members with the closest specialty to a problem physician are often
asked to evaluate the care, forcing them to juggle two roles—that of expert and
board member.[19] Many board members rarely challenge in-house expert
opinions because they have a long-term trusting relationship with the member-
cum-expert. The public members find themselves in a difficult situation when
the expert is also a panel member or staff summarizing the facts and offering a
rapid gloss on the case. Since boards rarely have members with similar
specialties, it is nearly impossible to elicit a second opinion, and questioning
colleagues without appearing to directly challenge their authority is difficult.

    A medical director presented a story with a long description of a baby who
died at birth. A physician on the board took the floor as an expert, saying
categorically, "It could happen to anyone—I vote to dismiss." The panel
concurred without comment. In this instance, no one questions the member's
authority to render a summary opinion or its substance; little discussion about
what happened or the standard of care may take place; and the public member
has little information to question the board member's expert opinion. The
board member's credibility—both moral character and expertise as a physician—
would be at stake if another board member asked, "Are you sure?" If one had
additional evidence, it might be reasonable to request a revision of
opinion, but questioning a board member's expertise without specific evidence
conveys lack of trust. This does not mean that arguments do not arise or that

public members do not ask for more in-depth explanation; it only means that rendering expert opinions may discourage opposing views and full-scale deliberation. Insiders often provide summary assessments rather than detailed and carefully reasoned analyses with a clear description of what should have happened, what actually occurred, and whether a reasonably competent physician would have done what the physician did.

Sometimes on boards favoring medical discourse, when a lawyer presents the case, and an outside expert provides a thorough report that is challenged, the problem is thoroughly explored so that a public member can understand what happened and what should have happened. Nevertheless, the doctors may still try to focus on why the doctor may have done what he is accused of. The public member, however, has the evidence needed to move the discussion in a different direction. Most boards use outside experts on some occasions. In the following scenario I developed, several patients were injured during surgery so they could not work. A lawyer investigated this case, reading the latest articles to understand the surgical process. Lawyers who handle medical cases frequently obtain considerable medical knowledge. She provided detailed descriptions about the usual practices and procedures, a long and careful description about what the outside expert saw from the scans before and after surgery, and a description of the relationship between what the expert saw in the films, what was written in the notes by the surgeon, and what should have been done. The expert report was detailed, clear, and intelligible. He stated that the surgery had not been done as was written in the doctor's notes (based on a comparison to the scans) and that the surgeries were incorrectly executed given the standard of care. The lawyer presented the case to the investigatory panel, which included a public member and two physicians, neither of whom was a surgeon.[20] The expert's written detailed opinion pushed the board members to question both his expertise and then to work to understand what happened when his expertise was established. The lawyer presents a legal frame:

> *Lawyer*: The result is we have several seriously injured patients after surgery, which were a direct result of the approach of the surgeon and confirmed in the expert's reports.
>
> *Physician Member 1*: The expert might be a competitor. He seems hostile. . . . He is not qualified legally as an expert as he may have know him.
>
> *Lawyer*: It is a large community and the expert is in a different area. He must have seen the name of the hospital on the film, but we have

already spent a lot of money. Besides, the question is not, "Was the surgery warranted?" but, "Was it done correctly?"

Physician Member 1: I'm not too concerned.

Physician Member 2: We can't ignore that the expert is one-sided.

The lawyer explains the surgery and scans step-by-step to the two board physicians. A very long discussion occurs:

Public Member 1: What the doctor who did the surgery said is different from what is shown on the films taken after the surgery?

Lawyer: What the doctor says he did is not what shows up on the postoperative films. The expert emphasizes that the surgery he did was out of date too. . . . This is not a vague generality but a very specific point-by-point abnormality. Look at the record, the doctor's report and the expert's report. Each one has a different problem.

Physician Member 2: I have a couple of comments. I will jump on the bandwagon. . . . We have an unbiased report, and he has stopped doing the surgery. He had a good rationale and needed a unique approach. . . . I'm second-guessing a surgeon. I don't understand this issue.

Lawyer: He shows poor judgment and outcomes.

Public Member 1: I can see that the film report shows that he did one thing, and the doctor's report says that is not what he did. He either wrote the report wrong or he was trying to cover up what he did.

Physician Member 2: I don't like the tone of the expert report.

Physician Member 1: It is not always black and white. . . . These surgeries cannot be defended but . . . documentation is a large part of the problem. There is no documentation in advance. It could have been a rational decision about why he took the approaches he did.

Lawyer: He said one thing, and the expert said another. . . . What he said in the operative notes is different than what the films indicate.

Public Member 1: I don't want him to practice on me or my family.

Physician Member 2: I have four questions. Was there an indication for surgery of any sort? What approach did he decide to use? What approach did he actually use? Was his report a mistake or a reconstruction? [These are fact-based questions, and they get the discussion focused on the evidence.]

Physician Member 1: We haven't talked to the patient. Was the approach decided in advance? What approach did he use?

Physician Member 2: The films and final postoperative report vary.

Physician Member 1: I will have to take the expert's word that he did not do what he said he did.

Physician Member 2: There is no evidence that he did what he said he did. And what he did was wrong. Did he say one thing and then changed it?

Physician Member 1: I don't know about reading operative reports, but what this says . . . I'm more convinced than I was.

Physician Member 2 (to Physician Member 1): Can you explain this?

Physician Member 1: I'll give it my best guess. . . . It is a similar issue. He claimed he did one thing and did something else. Why did he do these things? He's a good doctor.

Physician Member 1: The postoperative report, we should have a board member look at it.

Lawyer: What was done or not done is important—we need to trust experts.

No physician acknowledged that this doctor seemed to have little regard for patients except for the public member who said that he would not use the surgeon. Public members sometimes complain that the patients' perspectives tend to get lost even when they press them into full view.

This type of case is important for several reasons. First, the doctors, when they do not know the expert personally, often challenged the report and were hesitant to accept it. Second, medical expertise is relative; neither of these two doctors felt comfortable making an independent assessment. Third, nonphysicians, particularly lawyers who work regularly on medical issues, are able to understand technical aspects of cases, know much of the vocabulary used to describe treatment and diagnoses, and can explain clearly what happened and what should have happened when expert opinions are clear and detailed. And fourth, when the medical details of complex cases are carefully explained, public members can understand and engage in the dialogue.

Failure to Listen When Facts Are Provided by Public Members

With the medical frame privileged, public members may decide to go along and not raise questions that are likely to be dismissed. But they can also insist on hearing explanations or bring to the fore facts gleaned from documents to challenge a well-constructed story. As the medical coordinator addresses the incongruous facts that contradict the original story, the public member spotlights an alternative set of facts, but if others fail to follow the lead and explore the neglected information, the meeting will follow the familiar route. The physicians' minds are made up.

A medical coordinator presenting a case speaks for five minutes about the physician's illustrious career and the long course of treatment. But the doctor gave the patient a drug counter-indicated by one he was taking. The doctor claimed he was unaware of the allergy, and he suspended the medication. The medical director said that it was difficult to prove the effects and argued that the consultant wrote that it only "suggests" that the drugs affected the liver. What the consultant said was too simplistic, the medical director insisted and undermined the expert's point. The consultant was not in the room so could not explain his report:

> *Medical Coordinator*: There is a lot of good work in this area. I believe it is an oversimplification, but factual. I am sure there was a mix-up, and I can't fault the doctor. To me it was a minor impact.
>
> *Public Member 1*: But he gave the order over the phone, and there was the note about what he took. It was in the notes we received.
>
> *Medical Coordinator*: A mistake was made—the drug was listed in the notes. . . . He did a remarkable job with the rest in a complicated case and lots of work to benefit the patient.
>
> *Public Member 1*: How long was the patient in the hospital?
>
> *Medical Coordinator*: I don't think he was guilty of any transgression, and it was not a major factor in how the case was handled.
>
> *Physician Member 1*: No unprofessional conduct.
>
> *Public Member 1*: Yeoman's service was not the concern, . . . but I don't think he can be blamed. I support a letter of concern.

In my experience, public members do their homework and raise factual issues; the doctor, the public member thought, failed to look at the records, which implied some negligence and made a reasonable argument to which no one listened. And when he suggested sending a private letter to the doctor, no one was willing to do so, or look more closely at the record, or act as the patient's advocate. Glossing over what a public member says, especially when information on record is an issue, subverts a reasonable argument based on what happened rather than the doctor's background.

Trying the Patient's Story

When public members consider the patient's well-being, physicians may choose to acknowledge that focus, but the problem doctor's credentials as a fine human being may take precedence. To question a board doctor's assessment of character means questioning the judgment of a member as well as undermining trust. Doctors who examine patients of the opposite gender without another staff member present or carefully attending to proprieties can risk problems:

> *Medical Director*: A doctor treated a skin problem. The patient was critical of her care management. She said the doctor watched her change into a flimsy gown. He said he was busy with his notes and she says she didn't like it.
>
> *Public Member 1*: I accept the medical part. But the second about her distress, I am uncomfortable.
>
> *Physician Member 1*: I know him. He is a gentleman.
>
> *Medical Director*: He was surprised by the allegation.
>
> *Physician Member 1*: We should apologize for that woman.
>
> *Medical Director*: He is an established physician. It is a fact.
>
> *Physician Member 2*: I know him well.
>
> *Public Member 1*: I understand that. How can we encourage him to be more sensitive?
>
> *Medical Director*: Her distress may not have been apparent to him. He has no attendant. He says he feels badly.
>
> *Public Member 1*: He might want to take some classes in appropriate examination room behavior.
>
> *Physician Member 2*: It's a "he said, she said."
>
> *Public Member 1*: The burden is on him.
>
> *Physician Member 2*: He misread and was surprised.
>
> *Medical Director*: It isn't a typical "he said, she said."
>
> *Physician Member 1*: He has no history with us. He is highly respected. The patient is interpreting things differently.
>
> *Medical Director*: He knows it, and we don't know the meaning of the action. We don't have facts, we have two interpretations.
>
> *Public Member 1*: Should we tell him to take classes?

Each time the public member pushes the patient's side and stresses the impact of the physician's action, the doctors look for an alternative explanation and use what they know from the community. Pushing the argument further on the strength of the patient's word is hard, and requesting additional information risks undermining the trust among the board members.

The failure to pursue the patient's story is a common complaint by patients who resent that family members are rarely allowed to speak to the board. Occasionally complainants were invited to speak with an investigator, but board members tended to view their testimony as subjective and emotionally overwrought. Board members had stories of emotionally overloaded testimonies, particularly in hearings involving accusations of sexual misconduct where the alleged victims had to testify.

Patients' relatives are sometimes understandably very upset, especially when the mishap results in death, and want to talk to the board. Staff and board members explain that they find these situations difficult. A young man was not diagnosed fast enough to save or prolong his life. One board physician said that in retrospect the doctor should have diagnosed the problem sooner. The IC and medical coordinator in that scenario agreed to a conversation with a sister of the patient:

> *Medical Coordinator*: We understand, we think we understand. Just tell us. We try to determine unprofessional conduct according to laws and standards.
>
> *Sister*: I found lies.
>
> *Medical Coordinator*: We don't like it perhaps. Would you clarify? Did you go into the office?
>
> *Sister*: No, I wouldn't like to. The doctor called and asked me about some drugs. . . . My brother had a job with a big company and good insurance. The doctor canceled an appointment, but I called and he was free.
>
> *Medical Coordinator*: What happened?
>
> *Sister*: He went to the emergency room.
>
> *Medical Coordinator*: How long was it between visits?
>
> *Sister*: A short time.
>
> *Medical Coordinator*: All tests were normal.
>
> *Sister*: He would have wanted another test.
>
> *Physician Member 2*: Meanwhile he began to develop symptoms—we have to go by the doctor's notes.
>
> *Sister*: He was incompetent.
>
> *Medical Coordinator*: You need to prove that.
>
> *Sister*: You keep protecting yours from the people. Everything's a secret. Something funny went on and the doctor was lying.
>
> *Public Member*: I agree with Dr. ——. The doctor does the record at the time and you need to face the fact that certain things one says to a doctor he might not feel comfortable saying to you. He might have said something different to the doctor.
>
> *Sister*: He lied and you colluded. All doctors stick together.

Board members say they often felt uncomfortable with the emotional tone of patients and their families and may muddle the situation. Board members rarely express emotion toward each other during discussions of cases.[21] When board members let their emotions flare, it is usually after the hearing while reflecting collectively on the seriousness of the work and the difficulty of decision making at this stage.

Legal Discourse Can Change the Direction of the Story

The legal frame can effectively challenge medical discourse. Lawyers play increasingly important roles on boards. Several board members and staff reported that when a lawyer provides a legal argument, an alternative story may emerge, making room for fruitful discussion. A doctor who harmed several patients was reported to the board only after he objected to his hospital committee's recommendations. He gave up his license but was requesting reinstatement after completing a retraining program. The panel appeared to want to let him practice with supervision. The positive framing changed when the lawyer entered:

> *Lawyer*: You have to go to a hearing, or you can't let him in.
>
> *Physician Member 1*: A hearing would show he harms patients and took no responsibility.
>
> *Public Member 1*: I concur strongly.
>
> *Physician Member 2*: His knowledge was good, but he lacked judgment so I think he could work with supervision.
>
> *Physician Member 1*: I won't support him.

Lawyers used legal discourse to focus on, here, the need to hold a hearing. Once he did so, the discussion changed.

Despite a lawyer presenting a different argument than the medical director, some public members were captured by the medical way of defining a situation and did not take the opportunity presented to take the patient's perspective. Even when a physician board member and a lawyer tried to argue it was possible to see a case differently, the medical director's story had too much power over the public member. According to the medical director's summary, a patient with a heart problem made a complaint about his case management, but this physician's career was illustrious:

> *Medical Director*: She did a superior job managing this case. But she refused to send the forms to obtain workmen's compensation. She did not think it was her responsibility to fill out the forms and sent her very complete records instead. It's not unprofessional conduct, but we are very concerned about her behavior and could send her a private letter.

Board Lawyer: It is the doctor's responsibility to help a patient.

Physician Member 1: Could a person who is not an MD interpret the notes?

Medical Director: No.

Public Member 1: There is a case against a private letter—you need a real reason why and on what basis. Is there a rule?

Medical Director: Ethics are not based on rules; this pertains to quality of care.

Public Member 1: It is just a format issue.

Medical Director: It is a nuisance to fill out forms.

Physician Member 1: It is a denial of benefits, which the patient needs to live, and there is paperwork for everything, and it is sometimes overwhelming. The record was electronic, and she just sent it.

Public Member 1: I don't know medical ethics.

Lawyer: You need to meet the minimum standard of care.

Physician Member 1: The doctor's doing harm—it's a matter of principle. She is depriving the patient of financial benefits and needs a private letter. The doctor is taking her frustration out on a patient.

Limited understanding may lead public members to ignore behavior doctors define as unethical, and no expert established the standard of care here. Though the public member spoke up, he did not pursue the issue from the patient's perspective. The lawyer tried to establish that a standard of care must be violated to establish misconduct.

On other occasions lawyers, by discussing the evidence, push the board to consider the patient's side of the story. The panel tentatively accepted the staff's recommendation to drop the allegations, but a lawyer's intervention changed the direction of the discussion. An older woman complained that her doctor had inappropriately touched her and made sexual comments:

Medical Coordinator: The doctor was stunned by the accusation.

Physician Member 1: He came before the board after embarrassing his staff and some inappropriate actions with his patient before. The board sent him to therapy with a consent order.

Lawyer: There was misconduct. We took the deposition, and what she said he told her was she had a great body and stroked her. The doctor admitted he had said that but argued he was just joking.

Physician Member 1: I am troubled by the level of detail. It is too much to make nothing of it. He should know better. I think a confidential letter, but no unprofessional conduct.

Public Member: I concur.

The lawyer urged the board to see the case from the patient's perspective. Lawyers try to keep boards from straying too far from evidence and legal parameters, but lawyers do not always attend or intervene.

Legally Structured Investigatory Committees: Evidence, Violation of the Practice Act, and Winning

When legal discourse structures the review process, it clearly spells out grounds on which decisions are made. It requires thorough investigations to provide evidence. When lawyers and other staff engage in discussions, it brings multiple voices to the table. Much preparation is required both for staff to gather and for panel members to review investigatory materials before meetings—medical charts, interview summaries, expert opinions, and summaries of the cases. When cases concern negligence and incompetence, public members need to read the materials with special care, as diagnoses or treatments are not easy to understand. The materials are, however, sufficiently detailed for everyone to identify key issues and form questions. The panels typically have an option to dismiss complaints, require an interview with a physician staff member (not publicly reportable), or recommend parameters for a settlement (to be negotiated by a board attorney). If the last is not acceptable to the doctor, the case goes to a hearing.

As the focus is on the actions of the physicians and not character, board members do not see the doctors. Lawyers instruct medical coordinators and investigators to report only on what was said during an interview and to evaluate the evidence carefully to figure out what happened and then whether the actions of the physician fell outside the standard of practice. A written independent expert report or one prepared by a staff physician, or both, help panelists deliberate. The presentations include little information about the physician except education, date of licensure, specialty certification, malpractice history, and hospital affiliations. All who might know a physician under investigation recuse themselves and leave the room. The expressed goal is to identify cases that the board has a decent chance of winning at a hearing—an issue that sometimes provokes heated debate.

Lawyers frequently remind staff and board members to stick to the facts, to evaluate the evidence, and to ask questions. All are discouraged from bringing up matters unrelated to the physicians' questionable performance. If an investigator begins to outline the difficulties she had obtaining information from a physician, a lawyer can tell her to stop. The discussion that ensues revolves around the alleged behavior—what happened, did the action rise to the level of unprofessional conduct, was the available evidence sufficient to go to hearing, and would the expert testify? The terms used are "evidence," "facts," "winning a case," "statutory requirements," "efficiency," and "mitigation." The instructions to the panelists emphasize that they are to make their decision based on the act(s), not on physician character, which members knew little about. Occasionally, a more nuanced understanding of the doctor might arise from the investigator's report that sums up what the doctor said happened. Character could only be discerned from the investigator's report of what the doctor said, as the panel had no observational data and did not know the physician; any comments from investigators about the doctor's personality were disallowed, unlike the situation when the panel interviewed the doctor under investigation. Under a legally framed system, only evidence about what happened was supposed to be part of the decision about alleged misconduct.

Often staff and board members on legally structured investigatory committees engaged in spirited debate. A discussion of differences between what the IC panel received and the case as it would be argued before the hearing panel was important to anticipate, explained a lawyer, as defense attorneys would put on their own experts and witnesses and cross-examine the prosecution's experts. Lawyers want to hear the potential defenses, so they encourage arguments. A lawyer often argues the respondent's side of the story. Each side had its position forcefully articulated, in large measure because the staff did not want to waste resources with a weak case. All panel members had sufficient materials to query the investigators and the medical staff. When people expressed opposing views, public participation was also facilitated, as it provided more information and everyone could hear that more than one story was possible.

Members and staff argued their views. Sometimes the staff and panel had differing views; on occasion staff wanted to send a case to a hearing and the panel did not, and vice versa. Some cases had insufficient evidence, frustrating the panels. One such occasion involving a series of possible misdiagnoses I kept pushing, arguing about the public's vulnerability. I mumbled, "I know someone in that town. I'm going to have to tell him to stay away from that doctor." This may not have contributed to a rational debate as much as it expressed my frustration. A staff member frowned at me. A lawyer argued they had insufficient evidence given the statement of the outside medical expert. The lawyers' focus was squarely on the evidence on hand. I was unable to persuade others that patients' interests were endangered. The physicians on the panel followed the lawyers, who were afraid of losing the case. In the end, efficiency won.

Mindful of limited resources (efficiency), staff evaluated cases on probability of winning by finding misconduct. Legal and medical staff sometimes disagreed. A staff physician, incensed by a doctor's use of tests unrelated to the patient's complaint, first established what the symptoms were and then what tests were merited. He explained that this was not the way medicine should be practiced and meant that everyone's insurance would go up (patients' perspective), but a lawyer said that it was a waste of time and money to prosecute (efficiency) as only in one of the three incidents was a finding of misconduct probable and it was a low priority. A prolonged discussion about losing cases ensued—was it better to give a confidential warning or to prosecute and lose? Finally, two members decided that the risk of losing in a hearing was probable with only one reasonably serious event and settled for a private warning. The third member, a physician, wanted a hearing. Sometimes efficiency won over character questions. A physician might have lied on a hospital renewal form about a suspension, but it was cleared after he filled in the form of the second hospital. The physicians were concerned about his moral character, while the lawyers argued it would be difficult to win given these facts.

Staff lawyers know they might have to prosecute a case, and so they seek to get a good handle on all the issues involved and encourage public members to pursue their own line of questioning, which yields more food for thought. Arguments about interpretations of the facts help lawyers prepare for cases, as they have to anticipate the arguments from each side. In one instance, a panel and staff wished to know whether an action could be regarded as "gross" or "simple" negligence. Actions that rise to the level of medical misconduct vary among states, particularly as some states require "gross negligence" rather than "simple negligence" to prosecute. A debate ensued over a single incident and whether it was gross negligence. Once conflict among panel members demonstrated a lack of agreement over how "gross" the incident was, the prosecutors argued it was necessary to dismiss the case as "too difficult to prosecute." A defense lawyer, a board attorney argued, would be able to make an effective defense.

Establishing "gross negligence" hinges on law and medical judgment, but public members can weigh in as well. Whether one misdeed rose to the level of "gross negligence" was debated despite a prolonged argument in one case by a physician member that it did not. The debate started when a public member, fearing that a hearing panel might dismiss a single-incident case, argued that, while there was significant patient harm that appeared to demonstrate carelessness, she worried a panel might say it occurred too long ago. A comprehensive medical review of the doctor's more recent charts might find other incidents that would make it easier for a board panel to find "gross negligence" or multiple simple negligence cases—enough to prove misconduct. Staff thought additional cases were unnecessary, but the discussion then evolved into an argument over whether the evidence before the panel rose to the level of "gross negligence." A doctor sided with the public member.

Legally structured deliberations are often contentious, as all sides have a chance to air their case. "Sufficient evidence" is foremost on the panelists' mind. "Fishing expeditions" were discouraged. When a physician board member wanted to "see what was going on," when a young doctor clashed with his supervisor, a lawyer admonished him that this was not a good use of panel time since they had insufficient evidence to prosecute. The board member backed down.

Arguments supply everyone with multiple perspectives, pushing all participants to justify their positions. The conflict yields decisions that, while not always unanimously supported, result from robust deliberations. Only in the most egregious cases was there no debate. In such cases all had read the packet beforehand and were convinced by the evidence. One case, involving multiple sexual boundary violations, required no debate. The interviews with each alleged victim were carefully documented. The public member asked if any evidence of collusion existed among the alleged victims (answer—no) and if the women had agreed to testify (answer—yes), then said, "Revocation only," and the panel voted it to a hearing.

The more people present, the greater the diversity of views. With multiple views expressed, a public member has a better chance to ask informed questions and make an independent assessment and argument. In one case, a conflict arose between two physicians over "complementary" medicine. The public member learned from the discussion that the physician had given a patient "complementary" medical care but had not done the standard tests the symptoms required. The patient had a very serious undetected or unacknowledged illness. A committee physician volunteered that what often happens is that complementary medicine physicians say patients come to them for complementary medicine and see another doctor for conventional therapies. What this physician failed to do, a medical staff member complained, was irresponsible. The physician board member tried a more moderate approach, suggesting that medical schools were beginning to accept an evidence-based approach with complementary medicine. He compared it to homeopathy in the mid-nineteenth century when homeopathy killed fewer people than allopathic medicine. The public member asked whether the patient's chart showed that the patient had another doctor or had been referred to one to have appropriate tests. The public member had failed to look for this information in the patient's charts, for its relevance was not clear before the meeting. As it turned out, there was no such indication. Because of the failure to conduct standard tests and document that another physician also was following the patient, and, given the risks of not pursuing standard tests and treatment, the public member was persuaded that while the physician had the right to do alternative treatments, he should have done the standard tests or strongly recommended that they be done by someone else.

Physician characteristics may be used to assess possible mitigating factors in borderline cases but are discussed only after the panel has decided what the facts appear to be—and then, rarely. Although the "personality" characteristics of the respondent are never available, the years of medical school graduation are known. Age occasionally plays a role in discussing the disposition param-eters, but only after evaluation of the evidence. Some younger doctors are regarded as being amenable to remediation, in which case the panel may sug-gest a private warning. In one case, the failure to promptly diagnose a problem almost led to tragedy. A medical investigator who presented the case spoke to the difference between what the doctor should have done and what she did. The patient was sent home and survived only because he went to an emer-gency room. This was a serious breach of the standard of practice, but then the talk shifted to the physician's age and lack of experience. The interpretation by a board member physician was that the doctor had not learned to be "suffi-ciently suspicious." When the public member questioned the assessment of mitigating factors, the doctors argued she was young and had good training, and it was likely she could learn to be more suspicious of presenting symp-toms. The panel settled on a confidential verbal warning with a medical staff member to educate the young doctor about the severity of the failure. Here, the "legal" and "medical" responses reinforced each other. The language of law is "mitigation," and the medical response would be to focus on the physician.

When the medical and legal discourses clash, tension rises. The legal domain is not necessarily tougher on doctors—if the evidence is insufficient or the problem is not sufficiently serious, the case is dropped. In another case, staff presented facts relating to a young physician's "attitude problem" with health-care personnel. A physician panel member wanted a hearing "to get to the bottom" of what was going on and "to clear up" the situation, as the doc-tor was "well-trained" and young, but a staff member thought a hearing was a waste, as the offense was insignificant—it may have been poor behavior but not misconduct. The public member concurred. The legal response was that the offense was insignificant, but the medical response was that "he might be a problem personality," and research on the disruptive physician does show that "disruptive physicians" risk patient safety.[22] When the medical discursive domain or the legal/administrative discursive domain is the dominant frame, the public interest domain often recedes into the background. Legal discourse is concerned with evidence and law violation. Everyone has a voice here, questions are asked by all, people listen, and arguments are made by everyone. Yet the patient's perspective remains a secondary concern here, too.

A "Case Conference" or a "Probable Cause" Discussion?

Legal/administrative and medical/professional discourses produce different styles of case construction and discussion. The medical discursive domain resembles a discussion with medical peers about one of their own. Its form is similar to what can be heard in rounds and M&M conferences, where the goal is to insure that the doctors learn and understand what they might have done wrong. The medically oriented IC is only weakly connected to the following stage, legally structured hearing panels of, for example, Boards A and D. Board C's ICs and hearing tended to be more medically structured. The legally structured IC resembles a probable cause discussion that is preparation for a hearing organized by legal discourse where the review process evolves from the language and interpretations of the law and legal cases. While both discourses are heard on most boards, most tend to have one that more strongly shapes the deliberations during a particular period.

Some public members are more successful in engaging in reasonable debate despite the greater difficultly of doing so when discussions are structured by the medical/professional discursive domain. Public members manage to dig for buried facts, compose appropriate questions, and make independent assessments of cases. But when the focus is the character of the doctor and the "problem" is summarized and dismissed, they often do not have sufficient information to question the assessment and dismissal. Much depends on trust among board members. But sometimes board members may trust each other too much.

When a legally structured IC discussion revealed two conflicting accounts, the career of the doctor rarely entered the decision-making process, and public members had more resources to establish what happened in order to engage effectively in the debate. Open debate encouraged participation. Although evidence, facts, and standards of care do affect patients, rarely does one hear, "What about the patients?" at this stage.

In some cases, public members failed to participate not only because of discursive barriers but because they had been co-opted or lacked the skills of deliberation. The accountability advocates, who argue that public members make little difference, have reason for concern. It is not just the matter of a dominant discourse. Even in cases that do not require medical skills or much knowledge, some public members appear unprepared to engage in serious deliberations, evaluate what they hear, ask pertinent questions, and make forceful arguments. They appear to accept what doctors say.

Deliberative democracies depend on disclosure, on contest, on taking the role of the other, persuasion, and looking at decisions broadly. Everyone at the table needs to understand what happened and why they should be involved in the decision-making process. To shore up their legitimacy, boards need to justify their decisions by evidence and due-process fairness, rather than by a "trust me" argument. Everyone needs to hear the arguments and enough evidence and, while hearings are not always the best solution, private reprimands to encourage doctors to treat patients better need to be thoroughly justified.

The IC review is a critical stage in the disciplinary process. Most cases end here. As critical for public protection as this stage is, many members say there is little evidence that participants are guided directly by public protection concerns. Only sometimes does anybody ask, "Can you justify this outcome to the patient?" and "What can you say to the complainant?" The next chapter focuses on questions of transparency and the way it affects public participation.

Chapter 7

Hearing and Sanction Deliberations

Transparency and Fact Construction Issues

Only a small minority of cases, involving a wide range of behaviors (as described by Dr. Alan Schumacher, president of FSMB in 2000), are heard by a hearing panel, an administrative law judge (AJL), or a full board:

> A physician who offers fraudulent treatment to patients, sexually abuses them, or attends them under the influence of a mind altering substance has earned the attention of the state medical board . . . submit fraudulent tax returns, commit acts of spousal abuse, or be guilty of causing an accident while intoxicated. . . . To truly be a professional it is required that an individual have not only specialized knowledge and preparation, but also that one adheres to a special line of conduct or an ethical code. If medicine is truly to remain a profession, it must put the public interest above its own self-interest.[1]

Most "disastrous duffers," as described by George Bernard Shaw, settle their cases prior to hearings: "We may guess that the medical profession, like other professions, consists of a small percentage of highly gifted persons at one end, and a small percentage of altogether disastrous duffers at the other."[2] The general talk today is that of the public interest, but when settlements are negotiated by staff, board members may have little idea whether public protection or efficiency considerations were taken into account. Settlements save time, money, and court appeals but often result, in some states, in less transparency both to the board and public.

All hearings of Boards A, B, C, and D included defense lawyers, legally trained prosecutors, cross-examination of witnesses, recordings of the proceedings, and panel questions, and all used the "preponderance of evidence" standard.[3] But Board C held three or four hearings in public on one day before the entire board with a nonlawyer making legal decisions and Boards A, B, and D held hearings in private, over many days, before panels of three, including one public member, and advised by lawyers.[4] The short public hearings tended to wander from events in question, sometimes finding a general solution to a problem, but they were ill suited to developing facts in complex cases. The long legally structured hearings covered the events thoroughly during strongly contested hearings, highlighting conflicting accounts. Only Board C and the panel of Board B made findings of fact, established conclusions of law, and decided sanctions. When deciding sanctions, Boards A and D had short opinions from the hearing panels, which made it possible to interject the language of understanding, rehabilitation, and personal experience into deliberations, thus potentially decoupling decisions from established facts.

What is transparent varies significantly among boards, though all boards are more transparent than they were in the 1970s, when most worked in almost total secrecy. Transparency is not just a value in democracy, it is instrumental in creating public organization accountability and increases members' ability to make informed decisions. But transparency sometimes operates at cross-purposes; doctors' rights to privacy must be balanced with the rights of the public to understand board actions, to engage in debates about practices and policies, and to learn whether their own doctors are safe to practice. In some instances, public debate truncates discussion but opens other areas of debate and eliminates nonverifiable information. Decision makers also require transparency, both in evidence and in others' reasoning. As when corporate management controls information provided to public directors who make important decisions, some medical board practices and resources provide more information to those making decisions than others, and some members need more information than others, thus influencing debate participation. How to find a good balance between transparency and fairness to the disciplined physicians and the public is complex.

"Public" and "transparent" are not necessarily the same. Debates require arguments and reasons as well as facts. Although public decision making upholds the value of transparency, facts upon which decisions need to be made are not always transparent to board members, arguments and reasons given are sometimes truncated, and audiences are sometimes unruly. Long contested hearings in private are more transparent to those hearing the case, particularly with transcripts, and, if they also make the sanction decisions, may be more connected with the facts (as in Board B).[5] When a separate group makes the sanction decision with only a short opinion available, briefly listing the findings, what happened is less transparent to those making the sanction decision (as in Boards A and D). There is often less transparency when cases are negotiated prior to hearings. Sometimes no justifications are provided to the board, and only a short settlement announcement appears publicly.

When a sanction decision is made by a separate group from a fact-finding panel, with only a short fact summary available, board members may resort to assumptions about what had gone wrong or rely on personal knowledge of the reputation of the physician or interpretations based on the professional experiences of physician board members. When members began to discuss sanctions in public on Board A, it curtailed the addition of expressions of professional/personal experience, truncated public discussions of reasons, and required the public discussion of sad tales. Public hearings and sanction discussions do not have a clear predictive value effect on transparency and need to be balanced with privacy.

The Public Hearing before the Board

Multiple hearings on the same day heard by the entire board tend to be less contested than long hearings. The public hearings of Board C were often well attended and run by the board president, who made legal decisions. When I asked about the difficulty of making legal rulings without a law degree, a member explained, "We are well trained in legal issues and have a guide of definitions." The board discussed the findings of fact and the sanctions in private the following day, without a transcript, and issued short opinions. A staff member explained the process: "It is important to work towards efficiency—opening speeches should be limited to five minutes." He cited an out-of-town lawyer who talked for an hour and a half and lost the case.

This board also served as a counseling center. Staff and the security guard welcomed doctors on probation by name when they reported. In a waiting room, defense lawyers greeted staff while board members wandered in and out, speaking with waiting physicians. One public member said he spent time talking to doctors, including a neighbor, who was in a rehabilitation program for a second time. The phone rang continuously, and the woman answering the phone politely provided information to callers after checking on her computer screen. Board members worked to help problem physicians understand what they had done.

Hearings had the feel of a community gathering. Board members sat behind a large U-shaped table. The board chair sat in the center, and a board lawyer serving as prosecutor, the respondent, the respondent's lawyer, and the court reporter sat against the wall opposite the chair, about eighteen feet from most board members. Between twenty and thirty visitors listened at times behind one side of the board table. A staff member reminded the board that the visitors could see their computer screens. On some days they held four back-to-back hearings, but generally they held fewer than fifteen a year, as most cases were settled prior to hearings.

Construction of fact was often less than crisp. Lawyers' questions did not provide much structure. Board members took their questions in just about any direction, moving the discussion well beyond discovery of what happened. One case involved a physician charged with failing to arrive at the hospital for an emergency within a reasonable time frame. No experts testified about whether this was unprofessional conduct, and the board did not maintain its focus on the facts in dispute. Doctors who worked for the hospital testified about what they knew. The board president ruled on whether a statement was hearsay, while the audience, including hospital officials, whispered about the case. Aware that the town doctors were feuding, board members turned the hearing into a question about the practices of many of the town physicians as they struggled to understand the heart of what they saw as the problem—feuding doctors failing to serve the town well. Public protection was at issue, and the hearing structure permitted a broad range of questions.

When a public member tried to redirect the inquiry to the specific allegations, the doctors persisted with their lines of questioning. The public member tried hard to discover who said what to whom and why they did one thing rather than another. However, the questions continued to be directed more toward improving the medical delivery system for the town. The hearing morphed into how to solve a larger community problem. In fact, changing the physician culture in this town might well have protected the public interest better than a licensure action resulting from a more legally directed process about one physician.

Questions of character dominate many proceedings, and board members made every effort to give doctors a chance to tell their stories. Most respondents brought lawyers. One did not, but the board gave her ample opportunity to tell her story. She committed forgery before she asked for and was denied her first license in another state. Now she wanted a license in this state. Everyone sat listening intently, but when she asked staff to testify about their interviews with her, the chair said she could not ask staff to testify. The applicant kept repeating that since her forgery took place before she asked to be licensed, it shouldn't count: "I wasn't a member of the profession." Forgery and her refusal to acknowledge the problem indicated a character flaw, and the board, while listening sympathetically to her plea, refused her a license.

When boards found what they characterized as personality flaws, they were unlikely to support the physicians. A physician who had, in the view of the board, lied on his licensure application about another state's action was refused a license. He tried to excuse his failure to mention his discipline on his application, but his suggestion that the fault was not his but the other state board's did not help him. The applicant claimed that a media circus would have resulted from a hearing, but his argument ran foul of the fact that hearings in the other state were not public. Having established this fact, the prosecutor asked the applicant why they should believe anything he said. A public member asked if he thought he gave false information, to which the doctor responded that he gave what was appropriate. "I assumed it [the other state's sanction] was buried." A board physician informed him that the evidence from the opinion of the other state showed he was guilty and asked if the evidence against him in the opinion was false. His defense attorney argued that he (the doctor) understood it would be buried, that the offense had nothing to do with the practice of medicine, and that the young physician had no money and great credentials (the lawyer changed the focus from the act to the doctor's credentials). The doctor then blamed the public members in the state where he had been sanctioned and the cleaning staff who had testified against him who did not understand medicine (the activity in question demonstrated a lapse in moral judgment, not his clinical skills). His defense lawyer again tried to lead the discussion toward his excellent clinical skills and "superior" education, but the effort failed. The board decried the applicant's failure to reveal the sanction and to acknowledge the seriousness of the offense. Lying is an intolerable character flaw; good medical training did not overcome it. A board member explained to me afterward that if he had admitted his problem, he might have been treated differently. No rhetoric of rehabilitation was used here, the reason being that he failed to "understand" the seriousness of his lapse. The outcome echoed the language of public protection.

In another case, a physician failed to appear for his hearing on drug violation charges. He had been given two chances to complete a rehabilitation program, yet he did not kick the habit. He also made a false statement on his license application about a previous arrest. Despite his absence, the board prosecutor presented the case, and the board took his license. The hearings were too short to get many details. Little time was spent trying to establish or refute the credibility of witnesses or to build up the facts before making a decision. The attention fastened more on physician character than on what happened. The limited use of a legal framework permitted a broad range of questions beyond the evidence to establish what physicians did. As concerned physicians, board members wanted to get to the bottom of the infighting in a community and the moral character of the other physicians. The public nature of these hearings, also reported in the media, may have encouraged doctors to shape up. An administrator told me that they settled most cases because doctors loathed seeing their names in the news, even though the result was on the website. If reporters or community members were not present, little would be public as the descriptions on the website were brief.

Contested Hearings: Private and Transparent to the Hearing Panel

Legally structured hearings resemble trials; the prosecution presents its case, and the defense cross-examines the state's witnesses, after which the defense presents its side.[6] But after each witness and cross-examination, the panel members may ask questions. Administrative law judges or panels advised by lawyers decide questions of procedure, such as forms of questions, hearsay evidence, what can be put into evidence, and which witnesses may testify. In some states, prosecutors and defense attorneys raise questions of procedure more often than others. Legal considerations guide the process and provide more resources for all—even an expert's vita could be subject to debate—and, thus, transparency to board members is increased.

Board member questions contribute to the construction of cases. Members are instructed to use their knowledge to ask questions to develop evidence; that is, they are to use personal and medical knowledge to create a record. However, only on one board I know was it stressed repeatedly that expertise was needed to create a record by asking questions, not to assess cases independently of expert testimony. Administrative law judges or deputy attorneys general worked to ensure decisions were based on the record and wrote the opinions. Board B ALJs crafted very detailed opinions based on the panels' established facts and specific charges, which they did after hearing testimony and by reading transcripts and briefs (proposals of fact).

Orderly, contested hearings over several days with a panel asking questions of witnesses permit greater transparency than multiple hearings in a day, particularly for public members unfamiliar with medical practices and procedures. Knowledge areas mattered in the types of questions members asked, but the focus remained on what happened. In one case, a medical member's questions of a very technical nature took the respondent through the steps of the surgery in question. This strategy revealed gaps in the physician's knowledge that were then on the record and could be compared to what the state's expert said should have been done. A public member could not have asked these questions or assessed the responses, but with both expert testimonies and responses to the board member's questions, I was able to see that the physician had not followed the steps the state's expert considered appropriate. The defense expert's testimony was vague; I evaluated him as less than credible, and the panel physicians reached a similar conclusion.

The pursuit of details can increase understanding. A public member's naïve questions sometimes elicit information that more technical questions fail to bring up. I asked a respondent if it meant something when blood pressure was low normally and then rose during surgery as opposed to the situation when someone had higher blood pressure to begin with which then rose to the same point. The state's expert testified it was necessary to record blood pressures, but there was no evidence the doctor actually took vital signs. It was also clear to the board physicians when the doctor answered my question that he understood the importance of knowing a patient's blood pressure before surgery. The evidence of negligence was hard to ignore at this point, and the physicians continued to question him about his knowledge. Medical knowledge was important; it was necessary to have doctors on the panel who could ask specific questions, interpret responses, and ask additional questions to develop the record. Board prosecutors who try many medical cases learn medical language, but they cannot always completely follow through on detailed medical points or matters pertaining to complex hospital practices.

Nevertheless, in technical cases with medical terminology, public members paying close attention can spot contradictions. Less caught up in details of medical decision making, they may sense weak points in an expert's testimony. A fair number of cases include an element of psychiatric impairment. One case was complicated with many elements, including poor medical outcomes and possible failure to practice safely owing to psychiatric problems. One of the doctors on the panel pressed for the intricacies of the psychiatric diagnosis. A public member, standing back from a detailed analysis of a severe personality disorder, asked the psychiatrist what evidence he used to conclude the doctor was practicing safely. The response was, "He told me he was practicing safely." Since the panel had already heard experts testify about his unsafe practices, the defense witness's credibility was undermined. Such cases could be reasonably transparent to all.

When two experts address the board, all have to confront the possibility of two separate stories, and public members have a chance to ask more educated and pointed questions and make nuanced arguments. They can ask medical members for an explanation for why one expert was considered more credible than the other, and they may see things physicians miss. In one case, both the defense and state experts appeared qualified and credible according to their vitas and the reasonableness of their testimony. The physicians wrestled in determining which expert was more credible and asked the public member for his opinion. He suggested that the prosecution expert gave a "textbook" response to what the standard of care should be: "You must do x every twenty-four hours." The defense expert, using what the public member called an experiential approach, argued that a good clinician need not necessarily follow the "textbook" approach; if the doctor examined the patient and found no problem, then a physician need not repeat the procedure every twenty-four hours. The public member suggested that the panel need not decide between the experts, for the evidence that the doctor did the procedure or examined the patient every twenty-four hours was lacking. The two physicians agreed that it was reasonable to conclude the physician had followed neither approach and, thus, had not met the standard of care. Standing back and not becoming too caught up in the details sometimes helps to see what is going on.

Cases in which clinical and surgical judgments are necessary pose particular problems for nonphysicians, but sexual misconduct cases can be difficult for all. Desired transparency for what happened is difficult when there is only one alleged victim; the case rests on the credibility of the doctor and patient. Decisions get bogged down in "he said, she said" exchanges. Office staff may testify that they neither saw nor heard anything. No "material" evidence may exist; no witnesses may have seen anything, but the patient may have told people afterward. Decision making in these cases was often difficult, especially for physicians whose work focuses on test results and visual or auditory symptoms. The defense lawyer has room to develop strong alternative stories, impugn the character of the patient, or demonstrate the medical skills of the doctor. In one case, the defense attorney tried to impugn the character of each of several women who came forward. Only when a patient, testifying for the defense, described the problematic behavior as "comforting" did the panel begin to see the women's descriptions and inferences as plausible. They decided that what the women had described had happened. The panel then had to decide whether those actions constituted sexual misconduct. Using the FSMB's suggested standard, I argued that, if the women could reasonably perceive the acts as sexual, then kissing, touching, and sexual comments amounted to sexual misconduct. This case is telling, for it required the panel to see the acts from the patients' perspectives, which lent credence to the perception that the doctor's behavior was misconduct.

Judging the credibility of witnesses, particularly experts, is an important aspect of the discussion of what happened and what should have happened in competence and negligence cases and whether the event occurred in sexual misconduct cases where preponderance of evidence is the standard. When both the state and the defense provided experts to establish the standard of care, the panel was pushed to consider two different stories, had a chance to ask questions of each side, and had the opportunity to ask other panel members which expert they thought more credible and why. It made it more difficult to be dismissive of one side. Although the physicians may use their knowledge of medicine to evaluate the credibility of experts, public members tend to rely more on education, relationship to the problem doctor, and the clarity and specificity of testimony. Some experts were too closely affiliated with the doctors involved in the case (such as working together) or were not experienced in all the procedures under discussion. At other times expert testimony was very general, not appearing to bear on the alleged events, or experts appeared unprepared, making many mistakes and reversing themselves. Public members can understand these issues readily.

The process of developing a reasoned opinion, especially when transcripts and two briefs containing proposed findings of fact are available, as on Board B panels, facilitated transparency to all panel members who arrived with referenced transcript pages supporting their findings that related to each specific charge. The ALJs varied in the degree of specificity of fact they preferred, but all required careful fact construction. This process focuses the discussion on what happened, placing the evaluation of the physician's character in the background. It provides opportunities to develop an understanding of all aspects of the case and a structure for the panel to go about making its decisions. Reading the transcripts and briefs before the deliberations, I focused on questions that would help me understand the issues and that I could ask the other panelists. The preparations and discussions took time.

With full development of the facts, a clearer picture generally emerged as to what happened. Upon careful consideration of the testimony and briefs, one panel changed its mind halfway through the discussion and concluded that the prosecution had proved less than it claimed. They decided that the physician was responsible for the problems and that what he did was below the standard of care, but what they thought were two incidents of "gross" negligence and several others of "simple" negligence were really one incident of gross negligence and several of simple negligence. The process was facilitated by a collective reading of the transcript and debating the facts. The resources (transcripts of detailed testimony, briefs from both sides, and physicians who answered questions) were available for the public member to make a reasonable assessment along with the medical members. In the process of explaining to, and debating the evidence with, the public member, all had multiple opportunities to understand and to potentially change the assessment of the evidence.

When transcripts and briefs were unavailable, fact construction was more loosely connected to the testimony, for it was difficult to remember all the details of the testimony, and overall impressions were more likely used to make decisions, resulting in brief legal opinions. A member who took good notes and worked out an argument in advance of the decision-making meeting had influence over the outcome. During a very long case that took place over a period of more than a year with many witnesses, I prepared in advance of the decision meeting and had many factual matters laid out as I saw them. My arguments elicited only some counterarguments, and most of those facts became the basis of the opinion. Whether the construction was tightly linked to the testimony could be debated because we never saw a transcript, although the deputy attorney general who wrote the opinions did have access to one. Overall impressions, notes, and memories were critical in rendering the decision. Much happened between the days of hearing that could distort memory.[7] But with three members deliberating and recalling evidence, the panels probably made reasonable decisions. Having more information available, particularly in cases of clinical issues, permits meaningful public participation and for all cases provides more to discuss and increased ability to render a more detailed opinion for those who must decide the sanction.

By the time most cases get to a hearing, investigators have gathered a significant amount of evidence. But we need to bear in mind the trade-off between transparency and privacy in cases where patients need to testify, particularly involving sexual misconduct. Alleged victims of sexual misconduct are generally better off when they can testify in private, as it is difficult to get them to testify at all. But public transparency with the release of information after the IC meets, if the case is voted to a hearing, sometimes helps to build some cases by encouraging any additional victims to come forward, and, as cases take significant time before resolution, it does provide information to patients and other states.

Deciding Discipline in Public or Private

After the doctor is found to have violated the practice act, a decision about discipline is rendered that aims to protect the public, to ensure that the doctor does not harm patients. This is a difficult task as it requires assessment of the risk that doctors will repeat their actions. Character issues figure prominently at this stage, as Dr. Edmund Pellegrino pointed out, but the question persists as to how character is construed by board members.[8] To what extent is it evaluated on the basis of the individual's actions, board members' understanding of what the doctor understands, community knowledge of career history, and general reputation? The decision-making process differs when a panel hears the entire case over several days, and then decides a sanction, and when a panel hears the case, but the entire board, without the hearing panel, decides the sanction. When findings of fact, conclusions of law, and sanction are all construed and discussed by the same people, they become tightly linked, particularly with transcripts and briefs, and the public member has the resources to make assessments and arguments. The sanction decision is more embedded in the evidence of what happened. When the hearing panel includes different people than those deciding the sanction who have only a short opinion describing the facts, the disciplinary decision may be less connected to what was known to and established by the hearing panel. This is where the professional/personal experience of board members may come into play and where the presence of an audience may change discussion dynamics.

Although a basic tenet of a democracy, public discussion does not always increase transparency either to board members or the public. Public discussions may curtail "personal experience" arguments and eliminate discussion of information culled from places other than the hearing, but sometimes public discussion deters open expression of questions and reasons. The situation is further complicated when an audience is aroused and a breakdown in civility occurs. Board members, nevertheless, usually took the decision seriously, knowing not only that it will affect the respondent's career and be reported to the national and Federation data banks,[9] but also that their duty is public protection.[10]

Board structures that tightly link fact finding to disciplinary decision minimize the use of personal/professional experience rationales, as does public debate. When the board panel hears a case over several days and decides the findings of fact and sanction, the focus stays on the facts, thereby minimizing the use of members' medical experiences or personal standards of care in the discussions. Administrative law judges prohibit discussion of information not on the record and remind panelists that they must establish facts from evidence and evaluate the credibility of witnesses; little information is available about the character of physicians except what can be gleaned from observation of respondents at the hearings and what they did or did not do.

Although legally structured cases focus on what happened, participants still can take into account an individual's training, particularly when incompetence is at issue. How case facts are construed affects the disciplinary action, but the grounds for decision are what happened, not who the physician is.

If training was good, the errors that occurred may be judged as carelessness—the case is adjudicated as negligence, not incompetence. If it is judged as incompetence, the board might insist on retraining. In one case of negligence, one can see the different meanings attributed to actions: the public member argued the doctor's actions reflected not caring about patients, but other panel members saw him as taking on too many cases to make money, as financially self-interested. Based on their analysis, the panel physicians wanted to control the number of cases he was allowed to do. The public member wanted a suspension. They finally agreed the public would be protected with a short suspension followed by a restrictive order to practice only in a supervised setting. The interpretation of the facts mattered for determining what type of sanction might best protect the public.

Occasionally, cases raise a mental health issue in connection with the delivery of poor health care. The tension between rehabilitation, professional image, and public protection arises even after the facts are decided. In one case, the state presented clear evidence of significant patient harm; the defense put in evidence of mental illness. While all agreed about the facts of patient harm, one physician panel member focused on the psychiatric diagnosis and argued at the sanction phase for therapeutic treatment. I pointed out that the lives of several patients were endangered. They suffered severe consequences and revocation was warranted. The second physician stated that the doctor was a disgrace to the profession and agreed with revocation. Here both the patient and the profession's perspectives come into play. With the established facts of patient harm, two argued for revocation but used different frames. The public member took the role of the patient, and both doctors took that of the profession. Once the discussion focused on the facts of harm, the others persuaded the first physician. The focus on actions rather than the physician led to a different analysis.[11] Construing the facts of what had gone wrong and focusing on patient harm makes it possible for public members to make a strong argument from the patients' perspective. The focus on what happened provides the material for reasonable decisions.

When one group hears a case, establishing the facts, but another group decides the disciplinary decision, it allows sanction deliberations to stray from the facts, which opens the door to interpretations based on personal/professional knowledge. Doctors sometimes express sympathy toward a respondent by using their personal experiences to understand what happened. Public members can ask whether they would send a family member to the doctor, but they only occasionally succeed using this argument. If the doctor responds, "Yes, I would send family," the argument is over, as this is a professional judgment. The lack of transparency, particularly in cases that involve complex medical knowledge, gives the upper hand to physicians. Doctors have the authority of medicine behind them, and public members have insufficient information or understanding to challenge them effectively.

Closed sanction discussions sometimes allow observations and stories that are not in the record: comments about the reputation of the doctor, psychiatric diagnoses, and family issues. Discussions evolve into efforts to figure out why physicians did what the opinions say they did. It was easy to become caught up in such discussions, as I did on numerous occasions, for it is an interesting question why someone would do what seems like a strange or dangerous thing. Few tried to stop these discussions, and so these stories formed part of disciplinary decision making.

Since fact summaries are often short and vague, public members have little information with which to turn the discussion around. It is difficult in this situation to say, "Would he fail to do x again?" or "Perhaps he couldn't be bothered to let the patient know about the serious diagnosis." Without evidence from a prolonged hearing, excuses are easier to proffer; the story of the patient's suffering does not receive a sustained hearing. An inference might be that a flawed health-delivery system led to tragedy.[12] Reviewing the act from the physician's side, members may go out on a limb to locate exonerating circumstances. When no one thinks to or is able to argue from the patient's perspective, a public-protection discourse may not be considered.

A licensing exemption case illustrates the physicians' authority to define a case in terms of their own experiences and the public member's failed efforts to argue for the patient. Doctors sometimes get into trouble for prescribing regularly to relatives without proper documentation. A physician lost his license in another state for regularly prescribing narcotics to a relative over an extended period. He claimed he did not know his relative was an addict. The board physicians identified with the physician—anybody could be hoodwinked by a friend or induced to write a prescription for a family member without keeping a record. They talked for more than twenty minutes about writing prescriptions for family members and friends. Arguments about the length of time the doctor had provided drugs without keeping records and his lack of understanding of drug abuse were unpersuasive. All the board had in front of them was a short public opinion from the other state.

When a doctor makes a personal argument, it is also a professional judgment; physicians use personal experiences as rationales: for example, "We can't get it right all the time" or "I've done something like that." That leaves public members with little to say other than, "I'm feeling uncomfortable."

While an act may be poor practice, physicians often argue that it does not, in their view, rise to the level of "gross" incompetence or negligence, the legal definition in many states necessary to establish misconduct. The public member often has little specific information to make a cogent alternative argument. When a physician board member argues with a public member about whether an act constituted "gross negligence," physicians may respond, "It was a simple mistake, anyone could have done it." They frame it in terms of their professional experience. If public members still think the public is at risk and continue the argument, they are also criticizing the physician who claimed to have done similar actions. Many public members say that they do not know what to ask after a doctor personalizes a case. If they really believe there is a problem, they must think of ways to distinguish what the respondent did and what members say they themselves do. This is clearly difficult.

Examining an act from a physician's perspective does not necessarily lighten the sanction. Most doctors cannot identify, for instance, with a doctor who takes narcotics or lies. Sometimes the medical and public discourses arrive at the same conclusion while following a different path. In a case in which the physician lied on his license about not having a drug problem that was being monitored in another state, board members wanted to skip the discussion and immediately deny a license. They argued that lying was not permissible, they could not imagine taking drugs inappropriately, and he showed no understanding as he had already been given a second chance. Although the vote was unanimous, the public member's concern was that an addict who lied and used drugs was potentially dangerous to patients. Sometimes when doctors and public members spelled out their very different reasoning, they agreed on the sanction. More than one way exists to talk about any particular case or issue that comes before the board, and this is one way public members can contribute to the process of disciplinary decision making.

Decision makers owe others reasons for their decisions in a deliberative democracy. But public discussions do not necessarily reveal the "real or truthful reasons" and do not always work to encourage public voice or protection. Public discussion did limit the addition of ad hoc information and personal experience as justification. The transformation on Board A from discussing disciplinary actions in executive session to public meetings illustrates this point.

Deliberative democracies thrive on transparency, but public board discussions do not necessarily produce more transparency or better outcomes when it comes to disciplinary actions. Public discussions deterred informal information and lowered the use of personal/professional arguments, but they also often curtailed discussion. Pressure to open more board work to the public on

Board A did not immediately result in greater transparency or an increase in public protection. Few people attended public sessions, except when they had a stake in the outcome of a disciplinary case. But the television news filmed one early public disciplinary deliberation. In comparing notes afterward, we agreed that we had a difficult time talking about the case with cameras rolling, as we felt we were under siege. No one wanted to say anything, and when the discussion was over and the cameras left the room, the change in the atmosphere was palpable. Everyone wanted to chat. Public sessions made it difficult to ask what members thought might be naïve questions, especially with the press present, who often quoted liberally when a board member said something that might make a good headline. In some states the press and cameras were a regular presence. Most board members became reasonably accustomed to citizens and the press observing meetings, but they had to bear in mind that anything said could end up in the news.

While the audience may learn about the process, it can also make a fair outcome more difficult, especially if its members grow rowdy. In a case that first went to state court as a civil action against the doctor, the newspaper described the women's court testimony about his sexual activities, how his supporters showed up at the trial every day, and that 530 signed a petition to support him. A few more women came forward to testify at the board hearing after the trial finished. The board panel took more than a year to hear the case. The discussion about what to do with this doctor took place in public after the panel found misconduct.

When the "public" is really a number of "publics" and the case has received much attention, public proceedings may thwart the deliberative process. In the case described above, the board held the disciplinary discussion in a small courtroom with the board sitting in a slightly arced line in front of a judge's bench. The crowd, numbering almost one hundred, arranged itself on the courtroom benches. The overflow of press and the doctor's supporters stood all around the room surrounding the board and hissed every time the board talked about what the panel had found. A physician standing behind me mouthed nasty things about board members, particularly public members. Repeatedly interrupted, the board had a hard time engaging in an intelligent discussion. Protecting the public turned out to be hard to achieve when two hostile groups were backed up by throngs of supporters. Both sides were unsatisfied with the board's action, one because the discipline was too severe, and the other because it was not severe enough. The proponents of deliberative democracy could not imagine this public discussion as rational and balanced.

Another case illustrates a different complication that arises during public discussion. A doctor came before the board without a lawyer and, after accusing the panel of failure to grant him due process at his fact-finding hearing, insisted on retrying the entire case before the board at the disciplinary discussion. The doctor kept repeating "I haven't done anything wrong" and "If you were to understand the facts." The board members tried to explain that the board was legally bound to accept the findings of fact and that its role was to assess the conclusions of law and the appropriateness of the proposed sanction. Asked why he left his practice, the doctor replied that people were out to get him and that it was dangerous to stay put. Board members looked at each other, but no one wanted to discuss anything further. Finally, I made the motion to accept the conclusions of law and proposed revocation. In the parking lot afterward board members told me they feared the doctor.

Public discussion of "sad stories" presented a conundrum, especially with the press in attendance. One such case involved an elderly physician who had an exemplary career but could barely see and had endangered patients. He could not even see the board members sitting less than five feet from him. At the public hearing on his license revocation, he had trouble understanding that the board was not going to allow him to practice and kept repeating that he would only practice a little. Board members were afraid the story would appear in the newspaper and were relieved when it did not. This was a sad way to end a career. As this story suggests, some cases are more suitable for public discussion than others.

Several board members expressed deep concerns about debating disciplinary cases in public, yet the deputy attorney general insisted we had no other choice after a court decision about the state statute. A board physician explained that a sanctioned doctor had a recognizable psychiatric diagnosis that would have helped clarify his condition, but that discussing it in public was impossible. But the doctor's mental health status was not part of the case, and I pointed out that public disciplinary discussions were meant to prevent adding information not part of the official record. At the next public meeting the deputy attorney general made the same argument. We were going back and forth, with the press in attendance, when the board president finally said, "This is what the deputy attorney general says; we have to do it." All discussion stopped, but that did not totally deter some from bringing in new information from the medical community, although it was harder to insert facts not part of the official record in the context of public discussion.

Reminding board physicians about their responsibility to protect the public is reason enough to have public members on the board. Public members feel they have made a difference when they do not permit physicians to forget that the board's mission is public protection. After being asked about her feelings when she thought a sanction was insufficient, a public member at a national meeting replied:

> Then say so. Say what you think. Carry on a discussion. There are certainly times that we lose. What happens is not what we consider the desirable thing to happen. . . . I missed the last meeting. . . . I asked what happened and they said it was a good thing that you weren't there, you would have been really mad. It wouldn't have come out that way if you had been there. It was a case, a disciplinary case. I claimed it was a rape. He had sex with a patient, not one patient, but several patients. They [board members] decided in their ultimate wisdom that he was sorry about it and wouldn't do it again. I forgot what they did do but it wasn't what I would have done.

Sometimes it falls to physicians to remind the board that protecting the public is its primary responsibility. In a case, a board had the findings of fact and debated several theories for why the physician acted as he did when a physician finally said, "He hurt several patients and could do more. Isn't it our purpose to protect the public?" The public discussion stopped and the board voted for revocation. The disciplinary decision for board members is often emotionally wrenching, and public hearings make it even more difficult. Board members sometimes wait until the meeting is over to relieve the tension by joking and by rehashing the case, seeking to reassure themselves that they made a reasonable decision.

Transparency and Democracy

As Amy Gutmann and Dennis Thompson state, "It is not enough for people who exercise power over others to think that they know in their hearts they are right, because (1) they may in fact be wrong; (2) others cannot effectively judge whether the power holders are right or wrong if they do not subject their reasons to public scrutiny; and (3) others may reasonably regard them as less trustworthy if they do not offer their reasons publicly."[13] Gutmann and Thompson offer a clear rationale for open discussions among board members and for providing more public access to medical boards. Without transparency, boards cannot justify to citizens that they are acting legitimately, nor can others evaluate what needs to be changed to ensure greater public protection. What should be public is more problematic. As the previous discussion shows, debating in public has serious drawbacks, and certain cases may produce better discussions when shielded from the glare of the media and intrusive, uncivil observers. Yet opening up as much of the board deliberations as possible is a worthy goal to foster accountability and promote better practices. It also provides information for patients who must decide which doctors to use and how to improve board operations.

But there is a broader sense in which transparency is critical. Democracies need board transparency because their work is a public matter. As John Dewey observed almost a century ago, "If I make an appointment with a dentist or doctor, the transaction is primarily between us. It is my health which is affected and his pocket-book, skill and reputation." But because health care affects the general public, state regulation is necessary.[14] Much work needs to be done to ensure that physicians and health-care providers perceive boards as legitimate agents that will handle judiciously reports about problem doctors. Additionally, as part of the political process, nonphysicians and physicians need information about how the system works so they can develop informed opinions about how it should work. It is antithetical to democratic values and undermines the democratic process when the public has insufficient knowledge and information to hold meaningful debates. Lack of information discourages democratic participation and exacerbates mistrust of governing bodies. Nevertheless, assuring transparency and making proceedings public are not necessarily the same thing.

Despite the hope in the 1970s that public participation would increase accountability, mere presence of public members on boards does not automatically make boards more accountable or legitimate. Transparency is critical to all board members who often find themselves in unequal positions when it comes to access to relevant information. The cases that went to hearing on Board B were explored in depth with facts transparent to board members, but they were the least transparent to the public audience—except for their generally extensive legal opinions, which were posted on the Internet, making it possible to follow some of the panel's reasoning on points of law, evidence, and need for discipline. Board C held its few hearings in public, but most cases were settled, so that the board's reasoning on discipline remained obscure as the website posted only a short description of cases. With Board A, the public could hear a rationale for discipline, yet board members did not have detailed knowledge of the facts when they made their decision, and their explanations for decisions became less detailed in public. If no one attended the open sessions of Boards A, C, and D, little was transparent. But the provision of justifications for sanctions is essential. All board members need to understand all the cases and issues so that they can formulate questions and articulate reasonable positions.

While general public transparency is important to democratic legitimacy and accountability, how much information should be provided to the public is a matter of debate. The right to privacy is the value that has to be assessed against transparency. Court hearings are generally open to the public, and some are even televised, but jury deliberations proceed outside of public view, even though juries can in some states discuss their positions publicly after a verdict. The news media generally does not publish rape victims' names, even if the victims are expected to testify in public. Transparency also implies that information must be available to deciders so they can understand the case and assess what a reasonable outcome should be. Transparency varies in terms of what information decision-making groups have at their disposal and what will be made available to general public. Debating board matters openly keeps the community informed, but the presence of a public audience changes discussion, sometimes leaving "real reasons" buried under a pile of platitudes. "Public" does not necessarily mean transparent. Transparency and public discussions need to be balanced to ensure that the discussion does not lose its effectiveness, that board legitimacy is preserved, and that the right to privacy is honored.

Chapter 8

Democratic Deliberation and the Public Interest

For decades critics have wondered if letting professions police themselves was like allowing the foxes to guard the chicken coop.[1] The licensure movement unfolded under the banner of ensuring quality of service and weeding out bad apples within the profession—a public-minded rationale, to be sure, yet as this book has sought to demonstrate, community interests have not always prevailed in the course of self-regulation. While social closure greatly improved the practice of medicine, professional autonomy also helped solidify physicians' vested interests, which have not automatically aligned with the public good. The realization that doctors are propelled by self-interest as much as by community spirit has brought into the fray new actors—state legislatures, the federal government, public-interest groups, and the press; these new actors took it upon themselves to monitor the medical profession in the interest of the public. With new public and state agents in play, social control over the profession exercised by medical licensing and disciplinary boards has begun to resemble democratic politics in general, where outcomes depend on the skills, resources, and organizational assets of the participants. In this chapter, I argue that a deliberative democracy model of professional self-regulation offers a fruitful avenue for evaluation research and policy analysis and as a model for boards. The key issue this model addresses is how experts and nonexperts on medical boards can work together to safeguard the public good without compromising the quality of physician services.

In spite of claims of commitment to professionalism, doctors do sometimes act inappropriately. We know from numerous accounts that some use unnecessary procedures, regularly provide wrong diagnoses and treatments, commit fraud, abuse substances, commit acts of sexual misconduct, and decline to step in when they witness their colleagues' unprofessional conduct. Even today, some disciplinary boards see their role primarily in terms of rehabilitating errant doctors rather than guarding the public good. In the last few decades, however, the focus of social control in the medical profession significantly shifted from licensing and rehabilitation to discipline and protecting the public. In the last decade licensing has again emerged as a public protection issue. A broad range of public-interest groups and government agencies are now involved in national discussions on how to ensure physicians' competency over the life course for patients' health and safety. To articulate the deliberative democracy model, we need to start with the alternative formulations of social control over professions that sociologists have used.

According to Eliot Freidson, a prominent theorist in the sociology of professions, there are three common solutions to establishing control over professional work: (1) client control through market choices, (2) bureaucratic control with rules and regulations, and (3) professional self-regulation. Freidson is partial to the third model emphasizing professionalism, even though he readily acknowledges that professionals have often been self-serving; that professional standards have been challenged in recent decades under the pressure of market forces, consumerism, and bureaucratic control; and professionals have lost some sensitivity to being responsive to public interests. This is where a deliberative democracy model offers an improvement on the traditional model of professionalism by encouraging various publics to be involved with medical boards and other medical organizations that can speak on behalf of patients and forcefully advocate for public interests without turning the profession over to much more bureaucratic control or market forces.[2]

As our historical overview has shown, there were once voices opposed to licensure in the name of letting consumers and market forces decide who was fit to practice medicine. While we do not hear this argument repeated in its original form today—no one is advocating abolishing medical licensure—neoliberals frown on state regulation and are more content to let the marketplace weed out bad physicians. According to this ideology, a consumer is smart enough to choose a health-care provider for the price he or she is willing to pay (with some additional information) and to settle on one, including a provider who falls outside the realm of what is considered conventional medicine today. Radical consumerism also places choice in the hands of the consumer, who is trusted to shop around for sound information necessary to make an informed choice. Such claims are based on the notion that complexity is not an insurmountable barrier to patient choice, that intelligent consumers can glean relevant information from sources like *Consumer Reports*, and that forms of health-care that are not legitimized by the medical profession have merit.[3] Such optimism can be misguided; economists have doubts about information asymmetries and the consequences of poor choices in health care that can saddle patients unlucky with their health providers.[4] Even Adam Smith thought that some closure of professions was necessary to assure minimum competency among practitioners in a given trade.[5]

What undermines professionalism today, according to Freidson, is consumerism and bureaucratic control of health care, which manifests itself in the proliferation of guidelines, protocols, peer reviews, practice standards, and the emergence of rigid hierarchies in health-care management. For Freidson, these changes weaken a doctor's discretion and, thus, undermine professionalism. Any rational person, in his view, would look for ways to get around the rules. Economic incentives encourage doctors to milk either the payer or the patient by ordering unnecessary tests, using their own equipment that needs to be paid off, and making other commercial arrangements that can compromise the physician's judgment. Economic competition undermines professional social relations, which once promoted trust and goaded practitioners toward a normative consensus. Freidson leaves room for bureaucratic control and market forces in modern health-care delivery but only as a means "to reduce cost and control performance" and only insofar as these forms of social control "do not destroy or seriously weaken what is desirable in professionalism."[6]

The third logic, professionalism, is predicated on occupational control over one's work which, Freidson argues, requires social closure—licensure.[7] Such closure is not necessarily exploitative or conducive to domination. It allows professions to create educational and supportive institutions, career paths, ethical codes, common talk, and a service ethic, and it allows professions to develop and spread common knowledge. Professionals need to learn, practice, and identify with the community. According to Freidson, "The ideology of professionalism asserts above all else devotion to the use of disciplined knowledge and skill for the public good."[8] Freidson's sympathies are with this third pathway, even though his own research shows that doctors and patients sometimes have competing interests,[9] and doctors are hobbled by what he calls "clinical mentality" that encourages responsibility for one's own patients but not for patients treated by other doctors.[10] Professionals have not always used their discretion wisely despite codes of ethics, and yet repairing professional logic is the only way to control occupations where the work is exceedingly complicated, autonomous decisions are necessary, and expert knowledge is gained through long training. These hallmarks of professionalism

require closure provided by licensure and a service ethic attuning professionals to public good.[11] As Freidson states, "Practitioners and their associations
have the duty to appraise what they do in light of that larger good, a duty
which licenses them to be more than passive servants of the state, of capital, of
the firm, of the client or even of the immediate general public."[12] Even the fact
that closure promotes monopoly is not necessarily inimical to public good,
Freidson maintains, for it decreases competition among colleagues and provides disciplinary coherence.[13] In a democracy, he argues, people should be
able to regulate themselves—especially if they are expected to perform highly
technical work like that associated with the medical profession.

Autonomous professionals guided by a professional code of conduct may
indeed act as public trustees, but they are also likely to develop blind spots as
they are enveloped within a network of strong institutions where they are
trained, where they work, and that regulate them. In this traditional model of
professionalism, the physician is the ultimate judge of what is in the patient's
best interest, while the patient is more or less excluded from the deliberation
process. And the profession decides what is in the public interest.

My approach draws its intellectual ammunition from the model of deliberative democratic process articulated by philosophers and sociologists like
John Dewey and George Herbert Mead. These American pragmatists stipulated
that the public good is best articulated when all the relevant publics are
brought into play and when those participating in the deliberative process
learn to place themselves in the shoes of their adversaries or, as Mead put it,
"take the role of the other":

> The control of the action of the individual in a cooperative process
> can take place in the conduct of the individual himself if he can take the
> role of the other. . . . [This] makes it possible for him to take the attitudes
> of other individuals, and the attitudes of the organized social group of
> which he and they are members . . . so that he is thereby able to govern
> and direct his conduct consciously and critically. . . . Thus he becomes
> not only self-conscious but also self-critical; and thus, through self-
> criticism, social control over individual behavior. . . . The development
> of this process . . . is dependent upon getting the attitude of the group as
> distinct from that of a separate individual—getting what I termed a
> 'generalized other.'[14]

Thus, by seeing his behavior as others do, the individual will control his own
actions. This requires physicians to see themselves as the public does, and the
reverse.

Although Freidson sees "consumerism and managerialism" as undermining professionalism,[15] my research shows that social closure itself narrows professionals' perspective on public good and hampers their capacity "to take the role of the generalized other." Pragmatists are keenly aware of the barriers to adopting a public perspective in a modern society where groups are engaged in adversarial relations. Elite training and expert ideology endemic to professionalism differ from the exclusionary practices found in societies rigidly structured by class or caste, but the ideology of professionalism and expert knowledge may also discourage taking into account other perspectives and reaching a decision benefiting various publics. When professionals look largely to each other for guidance, they are more apt to confuse professional interests with public ones. Dewey and Mead clearly saw the dangers inherent in professional insulation, in setting up one's community apart and vigorously policing the borders from outsiders wishing to be part of the monitoring process. A strong medical community encourages members to treat each other with respect and follow local ethics, but this model of social control cannot escape the tension between self-interest and public interest, between collegiality achieved within the professional community and indifference and patronizing attitude toward outsiders. For example, collegiality has been invoked by doctors to justify not testifying in malpractice cases against their brethren. The mantra of "improving training standards" led to shutting down rival medical schools, impeding minorities, women, and financially strapped individuals from obtaining medical degrees and licenses, and limiting access of minorities and rural residents to medical services. Social closure has institutionalized a medical discourse that has inhibited intergroup communication and discouraged broadening the range of participants engaged in deciding the public good. The decision-making process is going to be truncated when the parties involved fail to take each other's perspectives, and such a process is going to backfire, as evidenced by the proliferation of patients' complaints, malpractice suits, and bad press besetting the medical profession.

Adding nonphysicians to the process of medical board decision making is a step in the right direction. Ensuring parity in deliberations involving professionals and nonprofessionals moves the process further ahead. Difficult as this task might be, it is not impossible. As I have shown in this book, there are ways to ensure that more voices are heard and heeded in the deliberations on medical boards. Adding nonphysicians improves the odds that public interests will receive a fair hearing. Interweaving legal discourse with medical discourse helps redress the imbalance of power. Challenging the ideology of professionalism that urges "independence of judgment and freedom of action," extols "collective devotion to that transcendent value," and demands *"the right to serve it independently* when the practical demands of patrons and clients stifle it"* will, in due course, make room for a more equitable and democratic method of delivering medical services and safeguarding the public good.[16]

Professional codes legitimize the doctor's autonomy and freedom of action,[17] but they also discourage physicians from paying close attention to patients' wishes and discourage the profession from paying close attention to the public interest. Institutions that have developed to protect patients' interests are now coming into their own, but they still have difficulties achieving their stated goal. We need to keep asking ourselves what encourages doctors to question and listen to their patients. Can one make reasonable decisions for others without effective communication with parties coming from different cultural and economic backgrounds? How can the profession decide what the public interests are when physicians tend to look largely toward each other? Does the fact that professionals sometimes act out of self-interest mean that the old-school professionalism is no longer tenable?

For a solution, we can turn to theorists of democracy, notably to Dewey and Mead. According to their theory, a society regulates itself though the discussion of issues by a diverse group of people who struggle to keep a common good in sight without disregarding the interests of parties involved. What this means is that we must put into place a framework for democratic deliberation that encourages all stakeholders to be part of the process.[18] Such a framework requires not only that diverse voices are given a chance to be heard but also that parties have adequate resources to make their case. Within such a framework participants learn to see themselves from multiple perspectives, think about their spouses, children, and parents in decision making, and take into account the needs of the poor, of rural dwellers, of diverse ethnic and racial groups. Encouraged to participate, people will be able to see others' views and take them into account when they are ready to vote and act. In the case of medical boards, this means including public members and inquiring how any decision will affect the various publics. For example, should a doctor who has been touching patients inappropriately and who happens to be a skillful physician be placed on probation, required to have a chaperone, suspended for a period of time, or have his license revoked? If the decision is not to revoke, is the probation system working? Can the board enforce provisions for chaperones? Or, for another example, will facilitated licenses for doctors practicing medicine over the Internet benefit the public? Is it open to abuse? What about granting additional privileges to nurse practitioners—is it a threat to patients' safety or to doctors' incomes? Will medical testing kits sold directly to nonphysicians through the Internet help or harm? These are the questions that implicate the public interest and that cannot be left solely to the discretion of professionals who may have financial stakes in the outcome.

Traditional peer review makes little room for the public voice, as was the case on medical boards. Courts and state legislatures pushed law and lawyers into the process, as public opinion demanded more action. Legal procedures challenge the medical discursive domain and provide additional resources for public members advocating public protection. It is partially this competition that permits public members to evaluate more fully what is going on and widens the range of stories allowed to be heard.[19] Competition, in turn, broadens power bases that affect the outcome and puts pressure on doctors to go beyond thinking that they are deciding purely technical questions and to consider a broader range of issues and values.

Of paramount importance, also, is that the public today is more educated and knowledgeable about its rights. Some patients now do a fair amount of homework before they decide where to get health care, which doctor to select, and what type of treatment to follow. Medicine practiced in two hospitals in the same town can differ substantially, with one physician counseling chemotherapy, the other taking exception to this approach. Who should the patient follow? Health care requires that patients be involved in making decisions. Greater transparency and wider information dissemination have increased patients' activism. The public is also getting more involved in new governance issues: discussions of continued competency, maintenance of licensure, and standards for reentry when a doctor has been out of active practice. Patients know there are doctors who fail to keep up, lose their skills, or violate the ethics of doctor-patient trust. That is why it is important for some of the public be involved in decision making and for all to understand how cases are decided on medical boards.

As medical boards decide whether professional work has been done appropriately, they rely on knowledge that is both nontechnical and technical, making it possible for the general public to understand much but also requiring evaluation by specialist physicians. According to Charles Bosk, "Moral failure is more often the subject of serious social control efforts than errors in technique."[20] Health care is a complicated process, and past failures are too significant and too important to let medicine be governed exclusively by the profession.

Democratic Deliberation

The democratic ideal envisions informed citizens with personal stakes in governance, deliberating on issues facing society, then voting on the alternatives and implementing the decisions embodying the will of the public. This lofty vision is hard to implement, especially in a modern society where knowledge required for informed decision making often exceeds the expertise individual participants bring to democratic deliberation. Group interests and private biases driving public debates further complicate the matter by fanning factional politics, benefitting some segments of society at the expense of others. Representative democracies tackle these problems by delegating deliberative responsibilities to elected representatives and establishing constitutional frameworks to ensure equal access to governance. To function smoothly, a representative democracy requires bureaucracy to service democratic machinery and enforce public will. Yet these bureaucracies "professionalize" and develop missions of their own, as happened with prisons in the first part of the twentieth century until they began to be challenged in the 1960s, when their powers and independence were gradually curtailed.[21] The greater the reliance on public servants, the greater the danger that bureaucrats will develop their own interests, thwarting the public's sovereignty. The challenge modern democracies face is to expand the room for public participation in a society dependent on civil servants and expert knowledge. It is in response to this challenge that civil society has spawned juries, school boards, community health councils, occupational regulatory boards, police/citizen review panels, liquor control boards, and parent-teacher associations promoting the public's involvement in governance. These civic institutions promote public participation in the decision-making process.

A substantial body of work highlights the critical role that democratic deliberation plays in sustaining modern society.[22] As John Dewey, a pragmatist philosopher and public intellectual, pointed out, "Democracy must begin at home, and its home is the neighborly community." His colleague, George Herbert Mead, agreed; democracies can sustain their vitality only by "passing . . . the functions which are supposed to inhere in the government into activities that belong to the community."[23] The spirit of Jeffersonian democracy informing these precepts is as uplifting as it is impractical in a society where administrators, professionals, and volunteers come to oversee and implement policy. The realities of the market and interest-group politics make state involvement in democratic governance necessary. These bureaucratic forms of control led some commentators to doubt the effectiveness of public involvement in a modern industrial society. Thus for Michel Foucault, public participation was little more than window dressing, a welcome opportunity for power holders to legitimize their control. Pierre Bourdieu grew equally disillusioned with democratic deliberation, which he came to see as something of a distraction from the political struggle led by the intellectual elite fighting to secure a bigger share of the public pie for the disadvantaged. Still, many theorists of democracy inspired by American pragmatism remain alive to the possibilities of public participation and deliberative democracy.[24]

Democratic deliberation is central to the operation of medical board activities, yet balancing community involvement, professional self-governance, and state regulations has proved a daunting task. History shows that left, to their own devices, doctors tend to police themselves in a manner that does not always coincide with the public good. The creation of Medicare and Medicaid prompted federal agencies and then state legislators to step up their regulatory oversight to ensure medical care standards and to keep costs down, with community members brought on board at this point. At first resistant, medical professionals on boards came to view public-member participation as benign, even beneficial, insofar as community representatives could be readily co-opted and used to legitimize their enterprise. It took time for public members to discover their voice, to take a critical stance. Lacking the technical expertise needed to challenge physicians, public members sometimes took the backseat and let physicians set agendas and lead discussions. Many today play active roles, but some lack the communication skills necessary for defending their positions, lack proper training to do effective public advocacy, and, invariably, are outnumbered by physicians. While some of these problems have been addressed in recent years, there are still barriers to public representatives' effective participation. The onus is not just on public representatives to learn proper deliberative skills; doctors also have to shed their blinders as functionaries in the medical domain and heed their community identities as patients, spouses, and guardians of the public good. This is why the query, "Would you send your child to this doctor?" can be effective, as it prompts a medical professional to don a different hat and exercise sociological imagination. Bringing legal experts into the disciplining process helps as well. Legal discourse allows different versions of the story to emerge, encourages the separation of documented facts from hearsay and a focus on what happened, and promotes due process. Legal inquiry may sensitize participants to the suffering of patients, present and absent—but not necessarily.

A central issue of deliberative democracy is how to get the public involved in the governance process. Electing representatives and voting in referendums on major policy initiatives leave the citizenry far too removed from daily politics, according to Carole Pateman. The participatory democracy model, she argues, has to reach beyond government institutions and elective politics; it has to empower citizens in the workplace as well, bring them into self-governance, and thus revitalize the citizen role.[25] Pragmatism-inspired theorists maintain that deliberations complement, and often prove more viable than, just voting or bargaining.[26]

The deliberation process on boards differs from the general policy debates carried out in such organizations as the Heritage Foundation, the American Civil Liberties Union, or Common Cause, which bring together those interested in specific policy issues and serve a particular constituency. These non-governmental organizations are voluntary associations; they articulate policy agendas and monitor compliance informally, but they lack power to enforce. Medical boards, by contrast, are constituted by state laws that charge their members with responsibility to oversee implementation of government regulations pertaining to the medical profession. Medical boards are hybrid organizations that bring together individuals with different backgrounds who are asked to review complaints, render judgment, and mete out punishment after collective deliberation establishes a violator's culpability. In addition, many boards are asked to make enforceable policy. The deliberation process is buffeted by statutes and regulations issued by legislative bodies. Stakes in board deliberations are high, and the consequences for the profession and the public are real. Hence it becomes important to ask how boards are constituted and how deliberations are structured.

In Pateman's model, a specified constituency (factory workers) must secure a place at the table, and discussions are presumed to be open and flexible, as expected in civil society. In the case of medical boards, however, one cannot escape selection bias; public representatives are appointed by politicians with particular agendas, as are doctors. According to Roberto Gargarella, it is the representation of "positions" in deliberation that is important, not the representation of specific groups.[27] How can we be sure that different views are fairly represented in the course of discussion? The disciplinary review calls for a limited number of debaters weighing in on the evidence, considering professional standards, applying statutory guidelines, and finally, voting to dispose of cases. Given this institutional setup, special attention should be paid to the question of who selects board members and how many public members are included. When institutions of governance are neither community groups nor government offices filled by elections or bureaucracies, it is far from clear who should be given a place at the table or how a particular member gets there. We do have rules for deciding who must show up for jury duty and who can—and should—be excused, but in the end, lawyers chose from the pool of would-be jurors based on who they feel is more likely to favor their client. That is not the case with when it comes to selecting board members or deciding what constitutes a proper mix of experts and lay persons serving on a board.[28]

Pateman's approach to creating citizenship is consistent with Dewey's and Mead's views of community involvement but is silent on how we should go about identifying eligible members. Even when membership criteria are clearly articulated, we encounter the difficulty of pressing citizens into service. Physicians join boards out of professional pride, duty, or self-interest; a citizen must be convinced to spend personal resources and volunteer for board work. Even when the selection process has been successful, we still have to see to it that participants are "free" and "truthful" in their deliberations.[29] The models of civic identity implicit in many democratic theories do not readily accord with the organizations like medical boards, which are made up of professionals, administrators, and public representatives. Autonomous, self-interested individuals claiming a place at the table as a matter of right are not always best suited for board work. Nor can we expect boards to represent all segments of the public or all medical specialties in equal measure. Some interests may be overlooked in a small group with limited resources and also committed to efficiency. Civic identity embedded in a small community within a larger one whose members pursue their own agenda is ill-suited for disentangling public from private agendas. And the problem is not just with the doctors pitted against public representatives—there are many "publics" with different perspectives and priorities.

We have to start by acknowledging that, in a diverse society,[30] community good is likely to be partial, that there is room for honest differences of opinion on matters of policy, and that each participant in a deliberative process must listen to various constituencies, cultivate multiple identities, and "take the role of the other." The more pronounced the ability to take the role of the other, the broader will be the "generalized other" that emerges in deliberations and the greater the likelihood will be that the outcome will be acceptable to stakeholders. Participation in public discussion creates competent citizens capable of inhabiting alternative perspectives and articulating an inclusive notion of common good. A key to this achievement is sensitizing all board members to the problems that the deliberative process poses for board members.

Inequalities are endemic and difficult to overcome. Even with citizens trained in assuming the role of the other and listening to multiple constituencies,[31] some groups gain advantage by using well-honed discourse, while others find themselves at a deliberative disadvantage because they lack communication skills and a well-articulated discursive framework to back up their positions. Members of the public are particularly vulnerable in this respect, for their interests tend to be underarticulated compared to those of physicians, administrators, and lawyers. Wielding a powerful paradigm gives deliberants an advantage. Many theorists acknowledge that the ideal of discussion free from coercion and open to all with a stake in the outcome is just that—a worthy ideal that is hard to achieve.[32] Insufficient research exists on how to equalize the power of the deliberants and specifically on how to empower public representatives in their struggle to get their concerns across without being overwhelmed by experts. We need a better understanding of how experts marginalize outsiders and what can be done to give nonexperts a proper say in the deliberative process. Broader public participation is part of the revitalization of the citizen role in governance, and it requires minimizing the power asymmetry that threatens to distort the deliberative process. Strengthening the discursive domain of law is one way we can begin to realize this goal.

There is no bright line separating civil society and the state; many hybrid institutions resist conceptualization. Thus we have prisons run for profit, federally funded welfare programs administered by private organizations, and a huge private security sector contracted by the military. Whereas medical professionals are adept at harnessing state powers to their advantage, they now have to contend with the increasingly assertive representatives of civil society who have learned to play the game and deploy legal arguments to ensure greater deliberative fairness.[33] Nevertheless, there is little discussion of participation and deliberation in hybrid institutions such as medical boards, which straddle the domains of government and civil society. Government plays a key role in medical board change, as it lays out a statutory framework that provides disciplinary tools and procedures, ensures some transparency, maintains membership diversity, and achieves court oversight. A strong civil society also needs a reasonably strong state; civil society needs the support of robust political institutions to fulfill its agenda and to balance the power of professionals, administrators, and the public.[34] This is a precarious balance at best. When boards are too embedded in civil society, it becomes easy for the profession to determine outcomes without other voices. However, when the balance of power shifts too much to the state, bureaucrats are apt to make decisions without much input from others and subordinate ethical concerns to the needs of efficiency and are subject to major funding cuts in times of state budget crises.

Deliberative democracy models offer few guidelines for balancing legitimacy, transparency, and public deliberation. This is a major gap in existing theory, for board legitimacy depends in large measure on the coverage its work receives in the local press and the publicity generated by public-interest groups. A critical issue is disentangling transparency from deliberation in public. Would more public deliberation increase legitimacy in the eyes of the profession or the public? Does increasing information flow increase legitimacy? As we have seen, deliberating in public has serious drawbacks in disciplinary cases where deliberants may hedge their bets, play to the media, or yield to the pressure from the party that did the best job mobilizing its supporters. Still, more information could be made available to enhance transparency and improve legitimacy of board actions both in the eyes of the profession and the public.

It is a challenge for a modern democracy to articulate and legitimize the common good. Media stories of physicians' misconduct and conflicts of interests have made the wisdom of second-guessing professionals clear.[35] State licensing statutes and government inactivity that permitted self-regulation failed both patients and doctors.[36] The era of complete self-regulation for the medical profession is over.

Overhauling the Medical Board System

The medical board system has been evolving for decades, yet the need for systemic reforms has not lost its urgency. Licensure and disciplinary practices continue to differ among states, making it difficult for doctors to obtain multiple licenses necessary for innovative strategies of delivering health care. The current system does little to assure patients that similar protective measures are taken everywhere. A physician whose license is revoked in one state sometimes can continue to practice in another state with a different set of rules. Many boards hold on to obsolete procedures, with legislators slow to make necessary changes. Board members still get insufficient training, little guidance exists on collecting data, and there are few clear standards for securing transparency and resolving conflicts of interests. The following recommendations are based on my conviction that effective boards require a diverse body of participants, improved data collection, formal training of board members, transparency balanced with privacy concerns, effective relationships between national and local organizations, and strong leadership from the FSMB in highlighting best practices and involving a broad diversity of groups in their discussions and activities.

Selecting Board Members

In most jurisdictions, the statutes establishing medical boards offer little guidance for choosing board members. States designate who is able to nominate board members, and some mandate a geographic distribution. It is left to the governors or their surrogates to figure out the eligibility criteria and the desired skill mix. Board physicians tend to be selected from medical society designees.

Sometimes the selected physicians had appeared before the board for discipline action. It is troublesome that public representatives may be affiliated with medical institutions, may work for medical industries, may be closely related to medical professionals, or might have been parties to multiple malpractice suits. It is the matter of concern, also, that states differ greatly on the ratio of medical professionals and public representatives serving on boards. In many states, boards lack policies designed to ensure that different groups have a foothold (with so few public members on boards, however, such a balance may be impossible to achieve). Few guidelines exist concerning desirable personal skills or qualifications. Often it is not a governor's priority; the resulting board composition may appear unbalanced, and the quality of membership uneven.

The need to ensure fairness and the general goal of strengthening deliberative democracy suggest the following imperatives and criteria for selecting board members:

1. highlight diversity, including regional, ethnic, and gender diversity, and various medical specialties among board members;
2. balance the ratio of medical professionals and public representatives on the board, with no less than one third from the community at large;
3. carefully explain the nature of board work and provide nominees with a realistic estimate of time they will have to devote to it;
4. vet all nominees carefully while weeding out unnecessary documentation that burdens board candidates; make sure to eliminate public members who are too close to the profession or have a narrow vested interest in a particular cause, physicians with multiple problems before the board, or doctors saddled with more than the average number of malpractice settlements for their specialty;
5. ensure that all nominations can be made from any source and that the nomination process is well known to the public;
6. specify the need for rotation among board members while ensuring continuity; and
7. educate governors and their appointment secretaries about the board agenda, membership needs, and the vital role public members play in protecting patients' interests.

Training Board Members

Boards are too small to be more than marginally representative, which makes it necessary for all members to think broadly as citizens and take the perspectives of various communities affected by board actions. With multiple communities and deep involvement in their own enclaves, all board members need training as citizens responsible for seeing issues from multiple perspectives. Training board members helps ensure that boards properly dispense with their deliberative responsibilities, that they are not beholden to a parochial perspective, that they partake in what Mead saw as the ever-growing democratic community committed to empowering individuals and groups previously excluded from deliberations. Board training will help its members develop a critical self that transcends the limitations of the present order.[37] According to Mead,

> The only way in which we can react against the disapproval of the entire community is by setting up a higher sort of community which in a certain sense outvotes the one we are in. A person may reach a point of going against the whole world about him: he may stand out by himself against it. But to do that, he has to speak the voice of reason to himself. He has to comprehend the voices of the past and of the future. That is the only way in which the self can get a voice which is more than the voice of the community.[38]

Training should sensitize all board members to the diverse interests they serve, the ever-present possibility of succumbing to a bias, and the need to advance the community well-being as the ultimate good. Board members must be encouraged to cultivate multiple identities and develop diverse skills. A well-designed curriculum would outline common communication problems, the negative consequences of stereotyping, and the high toll prejudices inflict. Both medical professionals and public members should be instructed on the limitations and strengths that each side brings to the deliberation process. All boards benefit from careful evaluation and articulation of its practices. Here are my recommendations for training a board:

1. designate a staff member to facilitate the learning process and outline the board mission, structure, procedures, responsibilities, division of labor, and lines of authority;
2. institute formal training sessions for all board members that include presentations, educational video shows, and simulation games modeling typical problems and situations;
3. bring new and established board members together to make sure the newcomers feel welcome and assign mentors;
4. periodically invite outside experts to update board members on best practices, latest legal developments in the field, and new challenges facing medical boards;

5. emphasize that the quality and effectiveness of deliberations improve when multiple voices are heard, when members with diverse expertise weigh in on a decision, when members listen carefully to others, and when each member learns to take the role of others; and

6. send board members and staff to Federation and CAC meetings, where they can learn and debate.

Data Gathering

Data help improve board functioning and transparency. In some instances board members do not have sufficient data to improve board functioning or even to make good decisions on cases. Board members dependent on administrators for the case-selection process are often troubled by lack of knowledge about the criteria used for choosing cases for review. Without enough data, the public has insufficient information to make decisions about which doctor to use or to understand what needs improvement in the process. To alleviate problems, boards need to develop data-gathering and data-reporting mechanisms. For example, boards should make a point of finding out who supervises doctors on probation and how to evaluate the probation process. Boards need to know who reports cases, particularly those likely to require investigation and hearings. Data gathering also allows boards to evaluate whether organizations that are required to report are doing so. Boards have to do more to encourage hospitals and other medical entities to report and explain to the public when the board can take action if few patient reports become fully investigated complaints. The following measures will help medical boards turn their decision making into a more data-driven process:

1. keep a log of reports that become complaints, break down the cases into categories (e.g., negligence, incompetence, ethical infractions, impairment issues, sexual improprieties, criminal violations, etc.), track changes, and look for patterns in reporting by different agencies and people (health-care organizations, government agencies, court holdings, patients, etc.);

2. inform board members about selection criteria for investigations, give reasons for excluding cases from consideration, encourage board members to go over closed cases;

3. match cases with resources needed to process them, balance the likelihood of prevailing in cases against seriousness;

4. track sanction patterns with an eye to increasing their overall consistency; and

5. make data and information public, but before doing so, engage in a discussion with the community about what it would like to know about board activities.

Balancing Transparency and Privacy

We expect democratic deliberation to be accessible to all interested parties, open for review, with outcomes publicly reported. This ideal is hard to implement in cases of medical board deliberations. Increased transparency has its own drawbacks. The reasons for that are similar to those requiring jury deliberations to be removed from public scrutiny (but in some states they can and do talk afterward).[39] Deliberating in the media glare can distort the process when members of the public misbehave or when board members feel intimidated by television cameras, but it does eliminate discussions of defendants' professional or private lives not on the record and makes reasoning public so the public can understand the process. Sensational cases tend to put extra burden on deliberants who may be swayed by biased media coverage or become afraid to speak. With free access to the disciplinary decision, there is a danger that one party may bring along supporters who intimidate others and disrupt the discussion. However, all should know how the deliberants reached their positions. Posting lengthy disciplinary opinions may pose fewer problems while improving an understanding of why doctors were disciplined and allowing the public to choose whether to use a doctor, for example, who is on probation. The board's visibility also may attract quality participants and alert legislators about its needs.

More and higher-quality information and resources must be available to members about how similar cases were disposed of in the past, what members' and staff reasoning is, and what the facts (technical and moral) of the cases are. This is transparency in a broad sense. Cases need to be transparent to all board members to allow them to make reasonable decisions.

But what is made available to the public varies wildly from board to board. Cases where sufficient evidence is available to hold a hearing for licensure action can be brought to public attention, for the public has a right to know if there is enough evidence to charge a doctor as dangerous to patients, as is done in some states. At this stage, boards need to be able to alert other states where the doctor is licensed that they may have a licensed doctor working who has been charged. Open hearings are less clear. Victims of sexual abuse might be less willing to testify in public, but the public and physicians might understand the process better after witnessing hearings, and doctors would become more aware of acts that might get them into trouble. Discussing sanctions in public may improve the quality of outcomes by curtailing references to what is not on the record. At the same time, such discussions can produce formal and cursory deliberations that make it difficult even for board members to understand each other's reasoning.

With these general considerations in mind, here are my recommendations related to board transparency:

1. select venues for meetings that can accommodate members of the board and the general public;
2. provide clear instructions on the code of behavior for those attending meetings;
3. hold well-advertised public meetings with discussion times posted and resources publicly available about new issues, such as scope of practice and maintenance of licensure (post publications, data, and summaries of the issues on the board website); personally invite groups who may be interested;
4. give the media as much information as possible to educate all;
5. respond to each report of a problem physician, and when the case is resolved, send a letter; tell complainants why their cases were not pursued or why doctors' cases were dismissed without discipline;
6. post detailed decisions on the Internet and send releases to the media;
7. make sure at each stage of the disciplinary process that the group has sufficient information, understanding, and reasons to make sensible decisions;
8. post statistical information on the website concerning the number of reports and their sources and the type and sources of cases that require hearings, in addition to how long the process takes;
9. make disciplinary cases public early to protect the state's residents and to protect patients in other states where a doctor is also licensed; and
10. educate both the public and medical groups about board activities and importance of community involvement in board policy deliberations and changing procedures.

Strengthening a Legal Framework

Boards operate under the statutory authority of a state. A state agency or, at other times, the board itself provides the administrative personnel, lawyers, and other resources that facilitate board deliberations. Board work is circumscribed by a legal framework that gives specified authority to its members and strengthens particular discursive domains at the expense of other discursive frameworks. In states with a strong legal structure, board members may be limited in the choice of cases that come for review or in what they can decide. However, a well-designed legal framework offers opportunities for deploying legal discourse, which offers not only due-process safeguards but also a way to talk about cases that may be lacking when medical discourse dominates board deliberations.

Board members are required to make judgments on different kinds of issues, from licensing and disciplinary cases to policy issues. People with different training and experiences bring to the table their own favorite ways of talking and deciding issues. Entrenched habits can be assets as well as liabilities. Doctors tend to focus on their peer's history and character, and only after they have gotten a feel for the problem physician do they shift attention to the incidents. Public members have to break some habits as well. They must learn to see beyond their own social group, pay heed to special needs of publics other than their own. The expertise all members acquired in the course of life and work may come handy in deliberations, and they should be encouraged to flex their expert muscles where it is prudent. All participants need to learn that they are not autonomous actors; everyone has to cultivate a civic identity attuned to a public culture and common good in addition to their particular identity as members of a parochial group.

Board members with different backgrounds and discursive preferences must operate within a common framework that draws out their civic virtues and improves the fairness of the deliberative process. To facilitate this objective, boards will need to do the following:

1. review the statutory framework governing board work, identify the procedures that are given precedence in a given state, and work to empower the discourses that tend to be shortchanged;
2. use legal counsel broadly and consult medical experts other than board members to write reports; describe what happened and what should have happened (standard of care) in cases of possible negligence or incompetence; implement due-process safeguards and limit the use of professional reputation in deciding what happened;
3. at the early stages of the investigation, focus on what happened rather than on the doctor's history and reputation;
4. advise all parties about the legal framework governing hearings, spell out the rights and obligations of all participants;
5. identify shortcomings in existing statutes and communicate board recommendations to the state legislature;

6. open and work to sustain lines of communication between board members and legislators; and

7. make sure that all the board members provide justifications for their decisions and understand the elementary rules of evidence and due-process requirements.

Strengthening Relations between Boards and National Organizations

In every field one finds organizations operating on the cutting edge and showing consistently good results, as well as those plagued by dissension, poor case management, and staff turnover. Improving coordination between the local and national organizations is one way we can improve the quality of medical board work. While too much bureaucracy and standardization may stifle local initiative and innovation, greater similarity of standards and procedures can benefit physicians and patients alike. Acceptance of one licensure standard and the use of the common application for licensing developed by FSMB would be beneficial. More standardization of disciplinary language and practices would make the assessment of best practices easier. Comparisons across state lines are complicated by a patchwork of incompatible laws and practices. The percentage of local doctors sanctioned by medical boards may reflect, among other things, the number or types of legally defined categories of misconduct; budget constraints; state involvement; disciplinary processes; the quality of local doctors; the quantity and quality of reporting by health-care providers, health entities and the public; standards of proof; the number or quality of investigators; or the number or percent of public members. Given this variability, one should proceed gingerly in comparing boards across state lines.

National issues and ideas need to be adapted to local environments, just as local wisdom should inform national models. Active participation of boards in the national debates with the FSMB and the CAC facilitates local acceptance and adoption of national models. Following the logic of Theda Skocpol's argument that the decline of associational structures linking local and national engagement created a decrease in citizen involvement, I suggest that boards encourage and fund members and staff to participate actively in national meetings. This facilitates the exchange of ideas and presses local boards to align their work with best practices and national standards.[40] The more understanding and trust boards have in each other, the more likely they are to develop consistent strategies to deal with doctors who have been disciplined in other states. Strong communications among organizations—both local and national—are necessary. Three groups are critical in this respect: the state, the profession, and the public. They can be at odds, but they can work together to improve board and professional practices.

Local autonomy makes it difficult to move smoothly through the twenty-first century. States need to look beyond their borders to coordinate standards and deploy research findings obtained by national organizations. Although a new credentialing service of the FSMB facilitates licensure, it is still cumbersome, as states maintain different criteria particularly for physicians trained outside the United States and Canada. Perhaps licensure standards should be the same, which would permit recognition of licenses of other states.[41] Maintaining multiple licenses may become increasingly complicated as some states begin to each establish new relicensure requirements.

As we strive to improve the lines of communication between local and national organizations, we might want to consider the following recommendations:

1. define categories of disciplinary actions that all states could use;
2. create a list of the most important aspects of board actions, structure, and process; develop and administer a short survey to allow board members to express their ideas;
3. invite experts in board development to assess the performance of a given medical board; identify the resources needed for the board to improve its work;
4. spell out best practices in medical board work, summarize the achievements of high-performance organizations, and use national organizations to disseminate knowledge about successful operations;
5. bring board members to the regional and national events sponsored by the FSMB and the CAC; provide resource-poor boards with subsidies for its members; and
6. work to make it possible to use similar standards to ensure continued physician competency through the life course.

Many of these suggestions have been implemented in some states as board members, public-interest groups, and legislators struggle to improve board practices. Boards evolve from legislative changes but also from new staff and members as they make sense out of their work.

Democracy thrives on active citizenry. It requires competent agents familiar with their rights and willing to exercise these rights. The state plays a part in creating an intelligent democracy by bridging a gap between isolated groups.

Placing citizens on the boards that regulate professions is one way it can achieve that goal. The state cannot stop there, however. It must do more to improve the board member selection process, encourage the training of participants, gather data, set up a viable legal framework, and coordinate the work of local and national organizations. All of these measures will ultimately promote democratic deliberations and improve the quality of life in our communities.

Conclusion

An Exercise in Democratic Governance

While bringing this project to a close, I did the paperwork required for my board reappointment. The process has grown more complicated in recent years, with extra forms and documents to produce. The change was made in the name of "good government," but it reminds us how difficult achieving the intended outcome is and how far we still have to go to achieve democratic governance worthy of its name.

Traditionally, board members invited to renew their appointments would submit letters of intent and update their vita. This time, attachments and forms sent to us were so massive they crashed my e-mail program. We were asked to supply high school, college, and graduate school diplomas, divorce papers where applicable, a complete list of publications and speeches, and all sorts of financial information. A state police officer, assigned to do a background check on every applicant, had to track down the diplomas that I could not find, even though there are no educational requirements for serving. It took me more than a day to fill out the forms and go to the governor's office for fingerprinting. The whole process seemed costly, intrusive, time-consuming, and unwieldy.

While the state examined aspects of my life that had little to do with my volunteer work, it did not bother to check for possible conflicts of interest. State bureaucrats did not care to know whether I was married to a doctor, whether I had a physician in my immediate family, or whether I am presently or was in the past party to medical malpractice suits. Given the hassle, it is hardly surprising that several valuable board members decided to quit rather than go through this unduly complicated process. Good government, you might say, has taken its toll. Concurrently, with states' deficits rising, many boards, especially those located within state bureaucracies, lost considerable amounts of funding and staff and took fewer disciplinary actions.

What these travails show is that democratic governance is complicated and that there is no clear blueprint for how to do it right. We can learn a good deal about democracy in action by focusing on the experience of medical board members. In this concluding section, I make the case that the history of medical boards teaches us not only about the evolving norms of the medical profession but also about American democracy as it continues to reinvent itself. By working together, medical board members learn to be good citizens as they improve the workings of the medical profession.

At the end of the nineteenth century, physicians and medical organizations got together in an effort to reconcile the practice of medicine with a larger public interest, and legislatures passed medical practice acts. For some physicians, medical practice acts and medical boards were an opportunity to increase professional status and improve market position; for others, it was a chance to rid the field of more egregious practices and abuses; for most, it was the combination of various, sometimes conflicting, agendas. The regulatory system as it evolved in the first seventy-five years of the twentieth century was predicated on the notion that medical boards perform technical rather than political or ethical tasks and that, consequently, the job had to be done only by specially trained people equipped with medical knowledge.[1] The technical skills required were certified by science, the latter understood as a value-neutral enterprise furnishing objective knowledge secured by disinterested experts.[2] While industry regulation was done by technical experts in bureaucratic agencies increasingly at the federal level, occupational regulation remained decidedly local. Doctors kept regulation within the local medical community, effectively controlling what doctors should know, who could become a physician, and which grading curve on entrance exams would properly delimit access to medical practice. Doctors bore the cost with licensure fees, and licensure belonged to the profession, with boards taking their cues from the medical community to ensure legitimacy. Such a system was as likely to protect physicians' vested interests as those of the public.

Although competing medical organizations grew apart over the years, the shared interest in keeping outsiders at bay pulled practitioners together. Accumulated strains within the medical community gave local state legislatures opportunities to assert authority after the federal government began to pay for Medicare and Medicaid. Board legitimacy became a public issue in the 1970s as outside groups began to weigh in on system shortcomings and offer suggestions for improvement. With government and public-interest groups gaining strength and the FSMB's financial independence, changes came from inside and outside the medical community.

In the 1960s and 1970s, Americans began to question the goodwill of the government, the competence of state bureaucrats, and the impartiality of experts. The democratic creed stressed pluralism and the power of participatory and deliberative democracy. Consumer groups waded into the political domain and demanded to be part of policy debates. Concerned with the profession's control of the market, the federal government took on boards and called for accountability, while declining to be directly involved in change. Local media revitalized participatory democracy by featuring stories about spectacular failures to regulate doctors. Encouraged by federal initiatives and media exposés of lack of disciplinary actions, legislators decided to act. This is when boards came under pressure to make room for public members. Some legislatures moved boards into state bureaucracies, while other boards remained independent in wielding their authority. Legal frameworks were strengthened, helped by court actions and statute changes, and boards devised new hearing and investigative tools, required more use of due-process procedures, and were required to open meetings. Board staff increased, as did their influence. Increasingly, nonphysician administrators run boards. In practice, most boards remained on the periphery of state bureaucracies, reflecting both the general skepticism of large-scale bureaucracies and the influence of professions. Some boards have added additional public members.

Communications between national and local organizations have steadily increased, even though local boards still hold on to their special practices. Some are tuned in to national debates; others pay less attention to what is going on in other jurisdictions. As board work focused on discipline, state courts were pressed into action, demanding that board practices meet legal standards. Their decisions did not work consistently to protect the public. Dangerous doctors were often allowed to practice while awaiting a court hearing, but the emphasis on the rules of evidence and open meetings had a salutary effect. Local mechanisms and interests continue to be decisive factors in determining the public interest.[3]

The fragmentation of medical organizations, which were critical to changes in medical boards at the end of the twentieth century, can be a problem when cooperation is required. Fragmentation complicates the debate about the need to update doctors' qualifications, with some medical organizations opposing new requirements as too cumbersome. How to measure knowledge and skills after ten, twenty, or thirty years of practice remains a contentious issue. A new system requires many organizations to sign onto it. Most states will have to pass legislation or change regulations to enable boards to add requirements for relicensure. Some have plans to do so, but opposition has already emerged. The public needs to be assured that doctors keep their knowledge and skills up to date and change their practices in light of new knowledge.

The story told in this book highlights communitarianism and scientism as powerful forces in a modern democracy. Those espousing scientism believe that experts armed with technical knowledge are fit to make regulatory calls, yet in its extreme form, the ideology of scientism has few adherents these days. The consensus is forming that it is imprudent to delegate regulatory decisions ripe with political and ethical implications to narrow, insular groups accountable exclusively to their peers. But the medical discursive habit of physicians encourages board members to think as physicians rather than as citizens of the broader community. While early boards wrote exams that limited the number of schools and physicians eligible to practice and disciplined doctors judged to be "different"—abortionists, drug abusers, developers of insurance plans—the public did not always concur with such judgments.

The medical landscape continues to evolve, unsettling those steeped in old habits. Medical procedures, the doctor-patient relationship, physicians' transactions with the state and the market—there is hardly an area of medical practice that has not undergone dramatic change in the last few decades. Treatment and diagnostic techniques change at an accelerated pace, the pressure to contain costs mounts, insurance companies become more intrusive, and government payments shrink. Patients are now more willing to challenge doctors about treatments after reading on the Internet or hearing advertisements. Others question the way we train physicians today. Some file lawsuits,[4] which, in turn, forces insurance companies to hike up insurance rates, unsettling established medical practices.[5]

Patients are often challenged by the practice of medicine. We now refer to the "preferred practice" as "patient-centered care," which means many different things: from receiving a survey (that one suspects enters the trash bin), to improved communications, to a medical team or "medical home" approach, or to better information. Patients learn that treatments vary from place to place, with little evidence to support those differences. Doctors either tell them what to do or leave decisions about treatment up to them with insufficient information to evaluate alternatives. Symptoms that arise after outpatient surgery often are inadequately described; it is difficult to know which complications are "normal" and which are not. Making one's own decisions may feel liberating, but it is also confusing and frightening. Medical information on the Internet tends to be written in technical language, and information featured on websites often doubles as advertisements for doctors or pharmaceutical companies who do not always have sufficient scientific evidence to back up their claims. Upset by bureaucratic decisions by their HMOs and insurance companies, patients must spend miserable hours negotiating for treatments and about their reimbursements—that is, if they have any insurance. Doctors have less time to spend with patients, and sometimes they choose to take their names off the insurance approved lists, forcing people to change doctors. Hospitals send multiple bills from different departments and doctors that make no sense to the patient. No wonder many patients are dissatisfied with the practice of medicine today.

Physicians have their own litany of complaints. Everyone appears to be looking over their shoulders and demanding more for less. Licensing boards are often awkwardly situated at the intersection of the public, state, and professional spheres. Accustomed to being judged by their peers in a fairly ceremonial fashion, they now have to deal with nonphysicians fortified by legally structured processes. Several groups express interest in making the National Practitioner Data Bank publicly available. The Federation and NBME have added patient-centered examinations for licensure that are graded by nonphysicians. Now the discussion is about demonstrating continued competency over a physician's life course and reentry standards after a physician leaves the active practice of medicine.

Groups interested in board work have evolved as well. The public, the state, the market, and new health-care providers are looking to exert their influence. More knowledgeable than ever, community activists complain to medical boards, urge them to update their policies, and seek direct participation in board deliberations. The media find board hearings a good source of newsworthy stories. Other health-care providers want to get a piece of the action that traditionally fell within physicians' scope of practice. Legislatures impose new regulations on boards, while courts require increased legal practices. For all these momentous changes, old habits are hard to break, and many traditional ways of conducting board business persist.

Looking ahead, we can see that reforms are coming, some well overdue. One urgent task is to improve reporting by health-care entities of doctors who exhibit patterns of errors and violate norms of medical ethics. Better reporting will improve health-care delivery, though enduring improvement will ultimately require fixing systemic problems. By streamlining board procedures according to a more national blueprint, one can obtain meaningful comparisons between boards and disseminate information about best practices.

We need to maintain a reasonable balance between the profession, the public, and the state, bearing in mind that too much state involvement risks the proliferation of ever-expanding bureaucracies and unwieldy regulations, that too much professional involvement threatens to marginalize public members and the public perspective, and that too much power devolving to the public can undermine the weight of professional judgment. Finding the proper mix for all these legitimate players and stakeholders will not only improve quality of health-care delivery in our society but also strengthen democratic governance in America.

Notes

Introduction

1. See Held (1996: 298–299).
2. OIG (1990).
3. Allsop and Mulcahy (1996); Becker et al. (1961); Bosk (1979); Freidson (1975); Rosenthal (1995); Stacey (1992).
4. In most states malpractice settlements must be reported to the boards, but each state has its own ways of handling these settlements. Many states have a system that triggers a review process once a practitioner has more than a specific number of formal complaints during a set period and with a particular settlement amount.
5. For a good description of several important aspects of how medical boards worked in general in the mid-1990s, see Jost (1997).
6. I did not include Guam, the Virgin Islands, or Puerto Rico, which are members of the Federation of State Medical Boards. Washington, DC, has its own board, and it is included in the statistics I provide in this book as a state. Doctor of Osteopathy refers to a physician who graduated from an osteopathic medical school.
7. One study of 2,013 households was commissioned by the FSMB (1997a).
8. This *Consumer Reports* survey was based on a national probability telephone survey of 1,026 adults, January 28–31, 2011 (*Consumer Reports* 2011).
9. In Britain the equivalent regulatory agency, the General Medical Council (GMC), created by the 1858 National Medical Act, has faced many of the same criticisms as the licensing boards in the United States (Allsop 2002; Moran 2002, 2004; Stacey 1992).
10. Researchers have argued over the origin of the decline in trust. Imber (2008) points out that the decline is embedded in the weakness of religion and growth of technical competence, while others insist that it derives from the structure and commercialization of the professions (Freidson 1986: 28; Larson 1977; Wolinsky 1993).
11. Schlesinger (2002) provides data that assess attitudes of elites and the general population toward medicine and questioning of medical authority in the mid-1990s, concluding that elites are less supportive of physician authority. The lack of support is related to belief in lack of medical efficacy, lack of altruism, lack of trust in the political involvements of the profession, and physicians' failures to act as agents for patients. Pescosolido et. al. (2001) argue that there has been some erosion of the public's positive view of physicians and those where the erosion is greatest are those who have the greatest stake in medical treatment.
12. See, for example, Saks (1995), especially chapter 1, for discussion of altruism and the public interest and Millenson (1997) for his discussion of the lack of scientific basis for many medical treatments.
13. Stewart (1999); Kohn, Corrigan, and Donaldson (2000). Many of Gawande's *New Yorker* essays were compiled in Gawande (2002, 2007).
14. More than fifty articles appeared in the *Boston Globe* and *Boston Herald* concerning the case. The two books were *Obsession: The Bizarre Relationship between a Prominent Harvard Psychiatrist and Her Suicidal Patient* (Chafetz and Chafetz 1994) and *Sex, Suicide, and the Harvard Psychiatrist* (McNamara 1994).

15. It is not my intent to define what is in the public interest but instead to examine how it is decided. See Saks (1995) for an analysis of the process by which he thinks that it is possible to arrive at what is in the public interest.

16. Ethnographers often change details of people's lives, construct composite accounts, and leave out the details that might identify participants, yet they present accurate depictions. This book is not about particular individuals or boards; it is about the different ways boards talk about and organize disciplinary processes. I heard repeatedly about every type of discussion I have developed here to illustrate variations.

17. Readers who wish to check the status of local physicians and how their state boards work can access individual board websites, which are listed on the FSMB website (http://www.fsmb.org/).

18. For a discussion of the importance of history to understand the present, see Garland (2001).

19. Stevens (1998: xix).

20. Black (1984) argues that we need to explain different forms of social control, which is a dependent variable with at least four formal styles: (1) punitive, which focuses on conduct; (2) conciliatory, which focuses on the relationship between the offender and the offended; (3) therapeutic, which focuses on the actor; and (4) compensatory. While Black sees them as separate, I found them all used within one organization and often articulated simultaneously. Most boards used either (in Black's terms) "punitive" forms, focusing on what happened, or "therapeutic" forms, focusing on the actor. Black argues that more law is related to punitive forms of social control than to other forms of social control. Garland (2001), however, focuses on change and the underlying shifting social structures and the need for new solutions to evolving problems of order.

21. A short history of the California medical board fails even to mention the ground-breaking change of adding public members (McCready and Harris 1995).

22. Abel (2011: 443) shows that lawyers worked for their self-interest in California as they developed their system of self-regulation. But he is interested in what the lawyers did in violation of professional ethics and why, not the process with which they dealt with disciplinary cases.

23. Expert or technological knowledge is what Habermas (1996) feared would become an ideology to justify social or ethical decisions.

24. "The most visible method of establishing something like an occupational monopoly lies in occupational licensing, a process by which a government agency grants exclusive official permission, sustained by law, to eligible individuals to work in a particular occupation" (Freidson 1986: 65). "Organized occupational groups have the exclusive right to determine the qualifications for particular jobs and the nature of the tasks" (Freidson 2001: 73).

25. McCleery (1971) included a critique of licensing boards, as did Gross (1984) and Grad and Marti (1979).

Chapter 1 — Public Member, Researcher, and Public Sociologist

1. Organic public sociologists work in close proximity with their "publics" (Burawoy 2005; Horowitz 2009; Wieviorka 2008); according to Burawoy, this happens only in civil society. I am extending this definition (see Brint 2005) to the uncomfortable state/civil sphere in which boards operate. Here my focus is on the interaction of the public sociologist and her publics (Wieviorka 2008), as a civic volunteer,

a researcher, and an activist. I am a member of the groups where I am an organic sociologist.

2. As described by Dr. Derbyshire (1969), a FSMB president.

3. Derbyshire (1969). Insiders include Ameringer (1999) and Stacey (1992).

4. The Federation started its own exam (FLEX) when the National Board of Medical Examiners (NBME) refused to test foreign medical school graduates (Derbyshire 1969). Since 1992 all new physicians take the three-part United States Medical Licensing Examination (USMLE), owned jointly by the NBME and the FSMB.

5. The Federation has argued for independent boards, in part for financial reasons, but while more state boards have reemerged as more independent, they are often short of resources. See Ameringer (1999) for an analysis and explanation of this push and success by the Federation.

6. Physicians can receive Continuing Medical Education credits necessary to maintain licensure in many states for attending FSMB meetings.

7. Starr (1982) argues that the profession has substantial social authority and also increasingly includes many forms of behavior as "medical issues," such as alcoholism and drug abuse (Conrad and Schneider 1992; Illich 1976).

8. Blendon and Benson (2001); Schlesinger (2002).

9. Several studies of patients show a more active and demanding public, and other studies show the importance of public-interest groups made up of people with particular medical issues who are demanding and knowledgeable about medicine (Haug 1973: 5; Haug and Lavin 1981, 1983; Rodwin 1994; Saks 2006). Freidson (1984) remains skeptical of the merits of Haug's data and analysis and sees little change in the monopoly of expertise and little loss of respect. However, Mechanic (2006) characterizes patients as "activated," showing what they know and demanding more.

10. In its most extreme form, unaware of the power of discourse, the public would add little to any discussion (Foucault 1973). Formal knowledge, such as medical knowledge, is seen as a threat to democracy, a tool for dominating or controlling everyday lives. This dominating discursive domain obviates the need for capture by the profession when the regulators surrender to the stakeholders (Stigler 1971); no alternative views are possible. The public members would not see the possibility that they might have different interests or ways of evaluating behavior than the profession; therefore, the vote would be unanimous and always on the side of the physicians. Co-optation where the public members do not think independently of the physicians is possible but assumes that the medical profession works to discourage the public from thinking differently and may be more or less complete. This view also requires that all physicians present the same perspective.

11. Chase-Dunn (2005) argues that public sociology is a stance within sociology and is evaluated both by external publics and sociologists.

12. I sent a survey to all administrators (sixty-six) in 1995 asking them when public members were added. Many did not know, and others were inaccurate when I looked at the statutes (forty-two responses). I did not use the responses.

13. In the case of Board A, the board moved its meeting to an earlier time, which allowed no social time, which in turn contributed to lack of interest in committee work or continuing for a second term. On Board B, the physicians generally knew other members from their hospitals and professional associations, but public members knew no one. It took several years to get permission to hold a public members' session at a training meeting that lasted only long enough for public members to introduce themselves.

14. See, for example, Bohman (1997).
15. Reason giving is often considered the most important aspect of deliberative democracy (Benhabib 1996; Bohman 1997; Cohen 1998; Gutmann and Thompson 2004).
16. I have added this criterion to try to resolve some of the real world issues of inequalities and diversity that raise the possibility of manipulation. This is one of the most difficult aspects of the deliberative process (Fischer 2009). Many of the theories of deliberative democracy assume that people need to be free of constraints to deliberate. But in the real world people are constrained by their own ways of talking about the world and tend to push those on others. They need to work hard to see issues from the perspective of others, and they need others to counter embedded perspectives. Hence, I argue for the need for a diversity of people and perspectives.
17. Whether and how emotions do or should enter deliberations is another contested aspect for proponents of deliberative models. On the one hand, some see the deemotionalization of public deliberation as essential (Habermas 1996; Hirschman 1997). On the other hand, others see emotions as an essential aspect of deliberations (Gambetta 1998; Goodwin, Jasper, and Poletta 2001; Nussbaum 2004; Shalin 1992). For an interesting argument about the need to deal with emotions that are tied to reason in complex manners in deliberations, see Fischer (2009). Those who see emotions as needed and integrated with deliberation argue that discarding insights from the senses makes for incomplete deliberative processes.
18. Many of the theories include the requirement of achieving "the common good" (Cohen 1997). Perhaps this is possible in the ideal world, but it is very difficult to achieve in the real one. One can work toward it and to consensus, but often it is impossible, and compromises are inevitable (Fischer 2009). Not only am I unsure how I would measure it, but I am not sure that it is achievable. Few decisions allow everyone to be satisfied.
19. Some people differentiate between procedural equality (are the procedures fair and give all the opportunity for voicing their positions?) and substantive equality (Knight and Johnson 1997), while others consider capabilities and resources as salient (Bohman 1997). Still others (Young 1997a, 1997b) consider some difference in perspective as a necessary resource for deliberation against the view that discussants must relegate differences to the sidelines (Elshtain 1995). According to Bohman (1997: 322), "The proper criterion for deliberative democracy is *equality of effective social freedom*, understood as equal capacity for public functioning." He allows for equality in standing and diversity of views in public functioning.

Chapter 2 — How Licensure Became a Medical Institution

1. Freidson (1970a, 1970b, 1986, 2001).
2. Some have turned the trait approach into efforts at sequencing those traits as stages through which a profession develops (Caplow 1954; Carr-Saunders and Wilson 1933; Millerson 1964; Wilensky 1964), but Abbott (1988) and Freidson (1986) have many critiques of this approach.
3. Wilensky (1964: 140).
4. Real estate agents, for example, have ethical codes, but many would argue that they are not professionals.
5. Happel (1901: 1302).
6. Rouse (1968: 76).
7. Caplow (1954); Carr-Saunders and Wilson (1933); Durkheim (1992); Parsons (1951, 1964); Wilensky (1964).

8. Berlant (1975); Freidson (1970a, 1970b); Gilb (1966); Hughes (1958); Larson (1977).
9. Dr. Samuel Hahnemann, the creator of homeopathic medicine, used "allopathic" to refer to "regular" physicians who became the "MDs" (Doctors of Medicine). It was considered a derogatory term. The "sects" or "irregular" medical practitioners refers to those who did not practice "regular" or allopathic medicine (Starr 1982: 100).
10. Starr (1982); Zhou (1993).
11. Zhou (1993) demonstrated through an analysis of the timing of licensure for thirty occupations that "person-sector" occupations predated "business-sector" occupations and that a strong state government enhances licensure for the person-sector but inhibits for business. This suggests that the power of interest groups does not necessarily overwhelm an ineffective state government.
12. Duffy (1993: 96–97).
13. Brieger (1972: 58).
14. Duffy (1993: 74).
15. Duffy (1993: 81–82).
16. Duffy (1993: 82–83).
17. Haber (1991: 184); and Starr (1982: 96).
18. Tennent (1734); Theobald (1764); Tissot (1765). See Cassedy (1991).
19. Gunn (1830); see Duffy (1993: 93–94).
20. Oldmixon (1741: 1:429), as quoted in Duffy (1993: 44).
21. Duffy (1993: 46).
22. See Dary (2008) for an analysis of the way doctors were paid.
23. Gray (1833), as quoted in Stevens (1998: 28).
24. As quoted in Starr (1982: 56).
25. Starr (1982: 51).
26. For example, Dr. James Still (1973: 81–82) was a mid-nineteenth-century physician who was advised by a lawyer to sell medicines in New Jersey as he was not a society member and thus could not collect fees for services.
27. Duffy (1993: 41–42).
28. Duffy (1993: 41–42).
29. Shryock (1967: 15–16) quotes this and gives the date as January 5, 1837/8.
30. Duffy (1993: 17–21).
31. Starr (1982: 118).
32. Stevens (1998).
33. However, many physicians were uneducated. For example, in 1850, of 201 Tennessee "physicians" who served a population of 164,000, 17 percent graduated from a "regular" school, 20 percent had taken a course of some lectures but had not graduated, 13 percent claimed to be botanics or steamers (irregular medicine), and 50 percent had no education in medicine except some reading (Shryock 1967: 31–32).
34. Stevens (1998: 29).
35. Licensing would permit requiring an exam that could necessitate more education and additional years of education.
36. Initial changes in medical education predated many of the state licensure acts. After the Civil War, several universities tried to extend the time needed for a degree and, at first, lost students. When in 1871 the president of Harvard, a nonphysician, decided to pay the medical faculty, lengthen the training to three years, and institute both oral and written exams, a few other universities (Pennsylvania, Syracuse, Yale, and Michigan) followed suit. Between 1870 and 1872 the enrollment at Harvard's medical school dropped by 43 percent (Duffy 1993: 205). The universities also

started their own hospitals in which the faculty could direct the clinical training of the students (Shryock 1967). In 1890 the National Association of Medical Colleges, renamed the American Association of Medical Colleges (AAMC), with a membership of fifty-five of the ninety "regular" medical schools, agreed to require entrance exams, a three-year curriculum, a six-month academic year, written exams, and laboratory work in chemistry, histology, and pathology (Duffy 1993: 207).

37. Millard (1887: 491).

38. Millard (1887: 493).

39. That the colonies sought to regulate physicians was not particularly surprising, for in England labor was regulated not to distinguish the "knowledgeable from the less knowledgeable" but to establish the state's moral authority over the labor force (Atiyah 1979: 67). The labor force was the object of significant regulation, including the Statute of Artificers that regulated apprentices (1563) and the Poor Law Act of 1601. Not only did the state regulate the length of apprenticeships, reserve the trades for the better-off sons, and require permission to move, but it also fixed wage rates. Some restraints on freedom were part of being a member of the society. A strong notion persisted within British society and was supported by the courts before the nineteenth century that a duty to fairness existed with or without evidence of a promise (Atiyah 1979: 147).

40. Duffy (1993: 39–40).

41. Duffy (1993: 43).

42. Fitz (1894: 8).

43. Abbott (1999) modified his ecological competition among occupations to include state and city politics. In an analysis of New York's nineteenth-century legislation, he demonstrates in this case analysis that contentious politics between the state and city levels and between political parties contributed to the licensing changes. Moreover, medicine was connected in various ways to the politics and through the public health movement.

44. *Hewitt v. Charier Jr.* 16 Pick. 355.

45. See Shryock (1967), chapter 1, for an analysis of early nineteenth-century licensure.

46. Shryock (1967: 34).

47. The formation of a national organization included "citizens interested in sanitation"; however, the organization's objective was to find experts to do the job, not to do it themselves (Rosenkrantz 1974: 58).

48. More (1999).

49. Barnard (1972); Duffy (1993: 14–19); Eaton (1972: 294–295); Haber (1991: 183); Rosenkrantz (1974: 60).

50. Some doctors, however, were concerned about the lack of technical knowledge of nonphysician members and wanted to exclude them from voting. John Shaw Billings wrote: "Further discussion of this subject in this Association, which is a mixed body,—not a body of physicians, but containing a large number of members who are not familiar with the technicalities of the subject, which is a purely medical one,—is injudicious and unwise" (from *Public Health, Philadelphia* [1882], as quoted in Rosenkrantz [1974: 62]).

51. Most cities took public health measures seriously by the end of the nineteenth century. Although some of the larger cities offered free vaccinations in the beginning of the century, they were not compulsory until the end of the century, and sanitary ordinances were not enforced. Some cities employed part-time nuisance inspectors and quarantine officials (Cassedy 1991: 57). Providence was the only city that had

: president of the AMA, advocated placing licensing in the
he hands of the medical societies, eight states initially put
the societies. The AMA also favored requiring state exams
push schools to meet minimal requirements if their stu-
xams became only one alternative pathway to licensure in
initial statutes passed (Baker 1984).

, Dr. Stewart argued: "No sooner, however, is one method
 than we find another. . . . Homeopathy, lately so fashion-
no resting place in Europe . . . took its flight across the
self in our soil" (Stewart 1972: 73).

 one pathway to licensure. Of the original statutes, forty
e avenue, twenty-four had an exam, thirteen named state
hip, and forty states included some years of practice in the
er to practice became the board-constructed examination,
ot become mandatory until the early years of the twenti-
Mississippi mandated one in 1882 and Wyoming in 1905,
1921.

byshire (1969) list Texas as having the first state board
) indicates that Wisconsin (1867) was, and North Carolina
9). Each state had its own strategy for regulation, and sys-
 different solutions generated as problems surfaced (Baker
tes, like North Carolina, had no provisions for sanctioning
 register or who failed to take an exam when they passed
.) credits the North Carolina licensure statute of 1883 as its
anged to require all who practiced medicine to be licensed.
written by Dr. Ivan M. Procter and Dorothy Long in 1959,
ry of the North Carolina State Board of Medical Examiners,
at in 1859 the state legislature passed an act that enabled
gularly graduated doctors" to elect seven members to form
to license doctors. Several of the doctors who were inter-
emselves members of the legislature. The legislature and
he public as gullible—"[he] will unhesitatingly commit his
and delicate organism to the hands of a blundering pre-
of its nature and operations is far greater, and whose mis-
ired" (Medical Society of North Carolina, 1852, cited in
3]).

nolsky (1996) found the first 466 applications submitted in
oplicants were women. In comparing older and younger
hat the younger applicants more likely to have had under-
ining after medical school.

.issing information on years of study, and eight licensing
g.

), the sectarians (nonallopaths) constituted about one-fifth
ans nationwide. In Rhode Island only a few wrote "do not

a perma
Boston,
Philade
most cit

52. In the ei
ety. The
a group
in 1904
member
50 perce

53. Stephen
some of
March 1
death ra

54. Dewey (

55. Between
where th

56. Seguin (

57. Bigelow
Treatise
was one

58. Erichsen

59. Weir (19

60. Duffy (1!

61. For a dis
Rosenbei
Dr. Whee
teenth ce
with dirt

62. Abel (2C
nineteen

63. Millard (

64. Stewart (

65. Stewart (

66. Friedmai

67. Starr (19:

68. James, B

69. Allen (19

70. Shryock

71. Cirn (198

72. For exam

73. Caldwell

74. Caldwell

75. When the
pected th
lation of
replaced
seven pec
the manu

76. Duffy (1993: 221).

77. Haber (1991:182).

78. Zhou (1993).

79. Starr (1982: 103).

80. Starr (1982: 107).

81. Although N. S. Davis, fir
hands of the state, not in
licensing in the hands o
for licensure that woule
dents were to pass. But
twenty-three states whe

82. Shryock (1967: 52).

83. In a speech to physician
of imposture on the war
able amongst us, findin
Atlantic and implanted

84. All states had more tha
included a diploma as c
medical society member
state. The strongest barr
but an examination did
eth century; for example
but Florida waited until

85. Shryock (1967) and De
(1873), while Baker (198
claims that privilege (18
tems evolved slowly wi
1984: 175–177). Some s
physicians who failed t
the 1859 act. Baker (198
first when the act was cl
In a history of that boar
One Hundred Year Hist
1859–1959, they show t
the medical society of ":
an examining committe
ested in this bill were
medical society viewed
own more complicated
tender, whose ignoranc
takes may never be rep
Procter and Long [1959

86. Aronson, Deary, and Ha
1895. Eighteen of the
physicians, they found
graduate degrees and tr

87. Six applications were
applications were miss

88. According to Starr (198
of the practicing physic

confine myself to any one practice" or "none in particular," and one Harvard-trained doctor wrote "eclectic/regular"). Several appeared unclear. Two University of Victoria graduates said "general," as did a graduate of the University of Vermont; a Starling University graduate said "medicine and surgery," while others claimed unique styles of medicine such as "electrotheraputics" and "Hygeiotheraputic."

89. According to Shryock (1967: 35), this school was chartered as a "water-cure" institute in the early 1860s, and it could give MD degrees with lectures in hydropathy and vegetarianism.

90. Of the first 350 license applications in Rhode Island, 14 were women, 5 of whom practiced homeopathic medicine. Several attended Boston University, which was, at that time, a homeopathic school and one of the few schools that admitted women. Most homeopaths in this state graduated from Boston University, Hahnemann, or the homeopathic School of New York.

91. Eclectics and their schools tended to be located more in the Midwest.

92. Requiring exams and increased years of schooling, which were added after initial licensing, contributed to the elimination of most other forms of medical practice and many schools, allowing regulars to dominate medicine.

93. Duffy (1993: 222).

94. Duffy (1993: 224–225).

95. North Carolina State Medical Convention Proceedings in 1849, as quoted in Procter and Long (1959: 1–2).

96. Stewart (1972: 64).

97. Bar associations, active early in the colonial period, pushed for educational requirements for lawyers. Though many were passed, they were difficult to enforce, as some judges did not support the associations, as they were not lawyers. The public remained suspicious of lawyers and bar associations, but lawyers were successful earlier than physicians in regulating their own as the Supreme Court said that the bar associations could and should regulate its members (Gallagher 1995; Haber 1991). They did not control the scope of practice (Abel 2011).

98. Dent v. West Virginia, 129 U.S. 114 (1889).

99. Hawker v. New York, 170 U.S. 189 (1898).

100. The legal challenges to licensure continued for decades. According to one estimate, boards received at least five hundred legal challenges to restrictive licensure in a fifty-year period from the end of the nineteenth century (Johnson, Dillon, and Henzel 2000: 116–122).

101. "Liberty of contract" at the end of the nineteenth century was contested, with some individual liberties upheld and with some actions that restricted liberties, such as licensure statutes, also upheld in the Supreme Court. However, even though Lochner v. New York, 198 U.S. 45 (1905), found that bakers hours could not be regulated to safeguard the public health, the opinion admitted that the state had police power to safeguard public health by having cleanliness rules. Judges may have been sympathetic to occupational organizations that wanted to carve out niches as the courts, too, worked to create a niche—judicial review over legislation—as legislation cut back on the court's ability to make social policy (Friedman 1965; see note 103 below).

102. Watson v. Maryland, 218 U.S. 173 (1910).

103. Friedman (1965) argues that the judges supported such legislation in part because of jurisdictional disputes with the legislatures. They were accustomed to making social policy, and legislatures had taken over that function. This position supports Abbott's (1988) argument that the professions solidify themselves in jurisdictional

disputes with other groups. But Friedman also argues that the courts supported middle-class and health-related occupations in licensure.

104. Kelly (1925: 5).

105. Kelly (1925: 45–46).

106. Kelly (1925: 6).

107. The first code of ethics of the AMA in 1847 served to symbolically isolate doctors and the public except in the doctor-patient relationship, where the physician remained in control. It denied that patients could be involved in their own health care: "Physicians . . . should unite tenderness with firmness, and condescension with authority, [so] as to inspire the minds of their patients with gratitude, respect and confidence. . . . The obedience of a patient to the prescriptions of his physician should be prompt and implicit." It was also used to claim professional status and monopolization (Berlant 1975).

108. Dewey (1954: 164).

109. Majoribanks, Delvecchio Good, Lawthers, and Peterson's (1996) research shows that medical competence in daily practice has been effectively challenged by law in the malpractice arena.

110. Additionally, the idea of what is covered by expertise and its relationship to the need for self-regulation is murky, as the amount and type of education necessary for all the different occupations licensed includes a wide range of length of study and of abstract knowledge necessary to do the work (Wilensky 1964).

111. Traditional views of professionalization were a series of steps (Millerson 1964; Wilensky 1964) or functions (Caplow 1954), and most even included licensing as a critical function or step in becoming a profession (Carr-Saunders and Wilson 1933).

112. Caplow (1954); Carr-Saunders and Wilson (1933); Durkheim (1992); Millerson (1964).

113. Ben-David (1963); Parsons (1964).

114. Dewey (1954): 207.

115. According to Rose (1999), communities are not generally made up of "natural" relationships; people have to be prompted to identify with the community, unlike the images of community in the nineteenth and early twentieth century. This is a much looser notion than that used by Goode (1957) in which doctors developed a shared identity, values, and definitions of interests. Although there was room for dissention and conflict, the core was deeply embedded. This notion of a tightly unified community was first contested by Bucher and Strauss (1961). Here I am using it in a looser fashion. Conflicts and heterogeneity are part of most communities, although some tolerate more than others. What that community is is debated: territory, strong social capital (Putnam 2000), natural moral bonds, or affect-laden relationships among groups of individuals (Etzioni 1996: 127) with shared norms, values, and meanings. Atkinson (1995) points out that functionalists tend to see more integration of "community," and symbolic interactionists see segmentation and conflict, but here I am referring more to the development by doctors of organizations to meet their needs as they arise and not to depend on others to solve their problems or allow them to contribute.

116. Freidson (2001: 78).

117. Stigler (1971) argued that, left on its own, the profession would control entry to its own advantage.

118. Derbyshire (1969: 44).

119. Ameringer (1999: 23–40) argues that state medical societies through their control of hospitals kept patients from problematic doctors: one had to be a medical society

member to join a hospital staff, and a society would not permit doctors who were incompetent to join. He argues that the antitrust case American Medical Association v. United States, 317 U.S. 519 (1943), which did not permit hospitals to exclude non-AMA members, created a gap in control of incompetent physicians. However, a doctor did not need a hospital affiliation to serve patients, and Freidson's (1975) work showed that doctors rarely knew about problems other doctors had despite working in the same office. I conclude that patients remained unprotected from problematic physicians, particularly those outside a hospital setting.

120. Shadid (1939: 165).

121. Shadid (1939: 165–167).

122. The federal government became increasingly involved in regulation in the twentieth century. Some efforts were overtly economic regulation, but other efforts, at least on the surface, were to protect the health and safety of its citizens. At the end of the Civil War, when Congress developed legislation (1865) to prohibit the importation of diseased beef, it was as much to protect the economic interests of the American beef industry as it was to protect the health of the people. Other early food regulation concerned products that could be substituted for the "natural" product in 1895 and 1896 (Eisner 1993). During the Progressive era, citizen's groups supported increased regulatory legislation. Nevertheless, many of the regulatory initiatives helped the industries as much as the consumers. The Pure Food and Drug Act of 1906 had the attention of many groups—Dr. Harvey Wiley, the chief chemist for U.S. Department of Agriculture, citizens' groups such as the Federated Women's Clubs of America; and the AMA. The AMA supported the act as drugs competed for consumer health dollars with doctors—not to improve patient safety (Eisner 1993).

123. Specialists needed general practitioners to receive referrals.

124. Duffy (1993: 224–225).

125. By 2000, in nineteen states only the societies could nominate board members and, in others, medical societies could still nominate most of the medical members, although physician nominees could come from a variety of sources.

126. Stevens (1998: 59).

127. Stevens (1998: 58).

128. Stevens (1998) argues that, in most countries, this function was performed by a government agency.

129. Stevens (1998: 58).

130. Stevens (1998: 64).

131. Flexner (1910). Several different views have evolved of the impact of the Flexner Report on medical education (Vevier 1987).

132. The number of homeopathic schools dropped from twenty-two in 1900 to twelve in 1910 and the number of Eclectic schools dropped from 1,000 in 1904 to 256 in 1913 (Starr 1982: 107). It should have been clear that medical boards were getting ready to increase educational requirements and institute state examinations of new applicants.

133. Derbyshire (1965: 64).

134. Shryock (1966: 32).

135. See More (1999); and Dary (2008, chapter 11) for analyses of the obstacles that women faced in getting an education and practicing medicine. For an interesting account of a nineteenth century well-educated woman who struggled to gain medical school admission and succeeded, see Vietor (1924). At the turn of the twentieth century, eight schools enrolled black students, but by 1923 only Howard and

Meharry Medical College remained with the help of foundation support. Only 93 black students were enrolled in white medical schools and 495 in the two black schools in 1947 (Stevens 1998: 71). Between 1904 and 1915, ninety-two schools either closed or merged until only eighty-five existed in 1920. This was in excess of the Carnegie suggested number of thirty-one schools (Stevens 1998: 68).

136. Stevens (1998: 66).

137. Derbyshire (1969: 62).

138. *JAMA* (1902a: 108).

139. Derbyshire (1969: 51, 55); and see JAMA (1902b).

140. Derbyshire (1965: 78).

141. By 1968 the board of the NBME included five representatives of the Federation, two of whom were on the executive committee (Derbyshire 1969: 47, 58).

142. Exams scores are now seen as the lowest threshold for admission into the profession.

143. Derbyshire (1969: 65–67).

144. In 1950 the Council on Medical Education created a list of recommended schools equivalent to U.S. schools but did it for only ten years (Derbyshire 1969: 139 and chapter 10).

145. The Educational Commission for Foreign Medical Graduates (ECFMG), initially created in 1956, certifies foreign graduates for graduate medical training in the United States. The commission has used several strategies to assess foreign medical school graduates (Derbyshire 1969: 145).

146. Derbyshire (1969: 164–165).

147. Derbyshire (1969: 34–35).

148. Records of the number of physicians sanctioned are very limited until the 1960s. The AMA and the Federation collected some state data on discipline, but no national record of discipline was compiled until 1984 when the FSMB set up a computer system and requested data from each state. Initially the data were not particularly accurate, as some states failed to send their records and others kept inadequate records (Derbyshire 1969: 77–78).

149. The articles appeared in the *Rhode Island Tribune* (1919, 1921).

150. FSMB (1921).

151. Eastman v. Southworth, 87 Ariz. 394; 351 P.2d 992.

152. Derbyshire (1969: 51).

153. As quoted in Derbyshire (1969: 51).

154. American Medical Association v. United States, 317 U.S. 519 (1943). For an extensive analysis of medical opposition to collective practice and insurance in the first half of the twentieth century, see Starr (1982: part 2, chapters 1 and 2); and Stevens (1998: chapter 18).

155. "The conclusion reached by some as early as the 1930's [was] that medical schools were over-regulated by AMA ratings and the requirements of state licensing boards." Some schools hoped that licensing would be returned to the schools to permit free experimentation with curricula and educational methods (Shryock 1966: 41).

156. The national associations were not always in agreement, necessitating trade-offs. The AAMC left the creation of educational standards to the state boards with each listing specific educational requirements for licensure. But the AMA, AAMC, and FSMB tangled, and the FSMB backed down, letting the schools set their curricula within local licensing frameworks and agreeing that its purview was fitness to practice (Derbyshire 1969: 166–167).

157. See Ameringer (1999: 15).

158. Derbyshire (1969). He also sent a questionnaire to medical societies and asked if they disciplined incompetent doctors. Only eight indicated that they did (Derbyshire 1965: 119). Also see Derbyshire (1966: 759).
159. Derbyshire (1969: 38).
160. Derbyshire (1974: 62).
161. President Kennedy's (1963) special message on protecting the consumer interest, March 15, 1962.
162. Berlant (1975); Freidson (1970a, 1970b, 1975); Gilb (1966); Haug (1980); Johnson (1972); Larson (1977); and Light (1991). Starr (1982: 13) argues that physicians "evaluate the nature of reality and experience[,] . . . the probability that particular definitions of reality and judgments of meaning and value will prevail as valid and true." This he refers to as "cultural authority." "Social authority," on the other hand, "involves the control of action through the giving of commands."
163. Forgotson, Roemer, and Newman (1967a, 1967b); Kinkel and Josef (1991); Roemer (1973).
164. Freidson (1975) found that officemates rarely evaluated or even saw the work of others. Earlier research on medical training (Becker et al. 1961) questioned the altruism of physicians.

Chapter 3 — Public Participation

1. Shaw (1957: 75).
2. For strong civic involvement, Sirianni (2009) argues that the government needs to become an enabler to counter the lack of social capital (Putnam 2000) or changes in associational structures (Skocpol 2002).
3. While underlying structural changes set the stage, several different results were possible as people and groups made choices and some groups had more power than others, but all had to give up something (see Garland 2001).
4. Medical services were more expensive to the consumer in part through control of information and by protecting the regulated group from competition (Benham 1980; Benham and Benham 1975; Friedman 1962).
5. Baggott (2002) documents some similar challenges in England. Allsop (2002) also found that the challenges were directed by the government in England.
6. What Parsons (1964, 1970) and even Hughes (1958) neglected in their efforts to understand the professions was the importance of the market; physicians effectively achieved monopoly control (Dingwall 1976; Dingwall and Fenn 1987).
7. McCleery (1971). In the 1960 campaign, President John F. Kennedy referred to the voters as consumers and in 1962 gave an address on the consumers' bill of rights. In 1964, President Lyndon B. Johnson set up the Presidential Committee on Consumer Interests (Creighton 1976: 42–43).
8. Williams and Matheny (1995).
9. Medical expertise was challenged by those in other health professions, who asserted that they were able to do tasks that physicians insisted only they could do (Witz and Annandale 2006), by developments in alternative and complementary medicine (Saks 2006), by increasingly expensive litigation (Dingwall and Hobson-West 2006; Vidmar 1995; Weiler 1991), by new and complicated forms of health-care insurance, by the increasing realization of the importance of knowledge gained from experience (Williams and Popay 2006), and by the spread of self-help groups (Kelleher 2006; Rodwin 1994; Williams and Popay 2006). See Brint (1994) and Haskell (1984) on expertise.

10. Berlant (1975) exposed ethical codes as promoting professional self-interest by for-bidding doctors from reporting on each other. Social control was supposed to be ensured through peer review, but Freidson (1975) demonstrated that physicians rarely conducted peer reviews, never criticized each other publicly, rarely knew about untoward events in their colleagues' professional lives, and only indirectly indicated when they saw something wrong with someone else's practice. Much was ritualistic even in hospitals and training (Bosk 1979). On licensing, see Forgotson, Roemer, and Newman (1967a, 1967b); Roemer (1973).

11. Creighton (1976).

12. Criticism from an economic perspective generally argues in favor of the free market and against licensing (Benham 1980; Evans 1980; Maurizi 1974; Wolfson, Trebilcock, and Tuohy 1980) in order to free the consumer to choose and force prices to decrease with more "sellers" entering the market.

13. A task force set up by President Richard Nixon in 1969 suggested consumer input into policy and programs and argued that health-care institutions had become increasingly self-serving (Bellin, Kavaler, and Schwartz 1972; Checkoway 1981a, 1981b, 1982; Chesney 1984; Klein and Lewis 1976; Schudson 1998; Vladeck 1981).

14. President Johnson used "maximum feasible participation" in 1964 as the rhetoric to encourage public participation (Rubin 1969). The Health Systems Agencies (HSAs) were developed by state agencies according to the 1974 National Health Planning and Development Act (P.L. 93–641) to make decisions concerning access to and need for health care and equipment. Although it mandated that 51 percent of boards be public members, most public members appeared to have little input, and their boards did little (Checkoway 1981b, 1982).

15. "Some managers are fearful of public involvement because they believe that it will reduce their power, open them to criticism, or just muck up the process" (Federal Interagency Council on Citizen Participation 1977: 12).

16. Creighton, quoted in Federal Interagency Council on Citizen Participation (1977: 44).

17. In 1970 an amendment to the Public Health Act (P.L. 91–519, Section 799A) directed HEW to report on certification and licensing for health personnel.

18. Vladeck (1981).

19. Little indication exists that the federal government wished to take regulation out of the hands of the professions or from the states.

20. Shimberg (1980); Shimberg, Esser, and Kruger (1972); Shimberg and Greene (1982).

21. Forgotson, Roemer, and Newman (1967b). In 1967, according to Shimberg (1972), there were twenty-five licensed health occupations. For example, Colorado first licensed dental hygienists in 1889.

22. Shimberg (1980: 165).

23. He remained active in the public-interest group Citizen Advocacy Center (CAC) until his death in 2003. I had several conversations with him about his work during CAC meetings.

24. The National Council of Occupational Licensing (state regulatory officials with a membership of about half the states) became more active, and states exchanged more information. Council of State Governments, National Association of Attorney Generals, and consumer organizations invited Shimberg to talk about licensing issues. The Conference of Consumer Organizations (COCO), formed in 1973 by leaders of com-munity and state consumer groups, organized a licensure conference in 1978 and included one session on public members. None of the speakers were public mem-bers (Shimberg 1980).

25. States asked for Shimberg's assistance at over twenty conferences. The National Council of State Legislators (NCSL) was given a grant under the Federal Inter-governmental Personnel Act to train state legislators about licensing issues, thus encouraging exchanges among states.

26. The HEW reports (Cohen and Miike 1973; HEW 1971, 1976 [preliminary and highly contested] and 1977 [final]) were produced in response to P.L. 91–519 (November 2, 1970) and included an amendment to the Public Health Service Act (Section 799A): "SSC.779A. The Secretary shall prepare and submit to the Congress, prior to July 1, 1971, a report identifying the major problems associated with licensure, certification, and other qualifications for practice or employment of health personnel . . . together with the summaries of the activities (if any) of Federal agencies, professional organizations, or other instrumentalities directed toward the alleviation of such problems and toward maximizing the proper and efficient utilization of health personnel in meeting the health needs of the Nation."

27. Personal communication, Harris Cohen, May 15, 1996.

28. The 1971 HEW Report uses Akers (1968); Derbyshire (1969); Forgotson and Cook (1967); Forgotson and Roemer (1968); Gilb (1966); Hershey (1969); and Rayack (1967) to support its critiques of licensing.

29. Cohen and Miike (1973: 241).

30. Cohen (1980: 304). Cohen's articles (Cohen 1973, 1975; Cohen and Miike 1974) in academic journals took a strong stance that licensing boards were extensions of the professional associations and developed not to protect the public from injury but to secure the profession's place in the world of occupations. Licensing boards sought public recognition and autonomy, thus making the state regulatory agency the public sponsor of the regulated interest (Cohen 1973:78). Cohen (1973: 79) used Derbyshire to criticize the medical societies' close associations with the boards. Although Derbyshire urged a single member (1969: 38), the effect would not have a significant effect according to Cohen (1973), who recommended a "substantial" number of public members. Derbyshire (1973) responded that highly specialized functions of the profession required that licensing rest with the profession—only the professionals can understand the ethical standards of practice (1973: 193). But he acknowledges the limitations of professional associations in providing the lists for the governor to appoint members.

31. HEW (1971: 28, 29).

32. Cohen and Miike (1973: 25).

33. HEW (1976; 1977: 10–11).

34. *ProForum* became *The Professional Licensing Report* in the 1990s under Anne Paxton's editorship.

35. Kelly (1925: 70). Kelly, in an extensive list of acts of misconduct, fails to mention incompetence or negligence, and Derbyshire (1974) found that only about fifteen states had "professional incompetence" as grounds for discipline and eight more had a category of "gross malpractice" in 1974.

36. Derbyshire (1969: 54).

37. Derbyshire (1976b), as did Morton (1976) in a position paper for the FSMB, expressed great concern for the involvement of the federal government in the proposed third report by Harris Cohen's committee. Moreover, the same volume of the *Federation Bulletin* includes a resolution of the Southern governors (Southern Governors' Conference Resolution 1976) to protest the report because of concerns with "states' rights."

38. Personal communication, Harris Cohen, 1996.
39. HEW (1977: 11).
40. HEW (1977: 14–15).
41. Riddle (1976: 3042).
42. Professional standards review organizations (PSROs), made up of licensed physicians, were initiated to supervise and evaluate medical service utilization by patients who received Medicare and Medicaid. This initiative to regulate physicians who received government payments was challenged unsuccessfully in the Illinois district court (Association of American Physicians and Surgeons v. Weinberger, 395 F.Supp. 125 [N.D. Ill.] [1975]). They are now called quality improvement organizations (QIOs).
43. The strategy of trading a possibility of federal involvement for public participation provides little indication that the AMA had lost influence.
44. Stein (1968: 53).
45. Hoffman (1973: 121).
46. Budd (1978: 131, 8).
47. Derbyshire (1973: 91).
48. Derbyshire (1974: 62).
49. Merchant (1970: 1950).
50. Edmondson (1971: 1855).
51. Morton (1975: 184).
52. Horns (1975: 82).
53. Memel (1977 :157).
54. Warshaw (1978: 322).
55. Morton (1980: 146–147).
56. John Ulwelling, executive director of the Oregon board, appeared on the cover of the *Federation Bulletin* in 1979 and was appointed to the federation board in 1981, but without a vote. The tensions between the federation and the executives continued through the end of the century, and in 2003 a discussion to make a voting spot on the board for an executive occurred.
57. Derbyshire (1976a: 384) wrote in a critical editorial, "The widespread curtain of silence, both of physicians and hospital authorities, causes problems in every phase of the licensing process." This was written after two significant cases (in New York and California) in which boards made headline news.
58. Freidson (1975, 1986).
59. One public member ran and lost (National Center for the Study of Professions 1981c: 2).
60. Wolinsky (1988).
61. Most would view the addition of public members as reminders to the public that the medical profession was accountable and working in their interest, thus legitimating physician authority and continuing self-regulation. Belief in physician expertise and physician cultural authority appeared to support the understanding that public members would be rendered incapable of taking an independent stance (Conrad and Schneider 1992; Foucault 1973; Illich 1976). The profession still controlled licensing through AMA committees, state medical society nominations, and exams written by the profession. It believed it was vulnerable on boards only in the area of a few errant physicians who might be taken out of practice. Only the deprofessionalization argument (Haug 1973) might support a position that public members might be anything but ceremonial.
62. Judicial Council of the AMA (1970: 588).

63. Gardner (1980: 361, 3).
64. This same argument is made for law (Wolfram 1978).
65. Derber, Schwartz, and Magrass (1990); Freidson (1970a, 1970b); Larson (1977, 1984).
66. Conrad and Schneider (1992); Foucault (1973); Johnson (1995).
67. Derbyshire (1969: 77–78).
68. Morrow (1985) documents the start of the impaired physicians committees. The committees perceived doctors as nonculpable—not responsible for their impairment—and were committed to rehabilitation and reintegration. The committees were run by colleagues and excluded the public. Morrow does not, however, see the programs as a response to the public exposure of medical boards.
69. The Federation conducted a survey in October 1993 with the initiation of the Ad Hoc Committee on Physician Impairment (1994). Of the 70 percent of medical boards that responded, 20 percent included sexual misconduct as impairment. Eighty-nine percent had an impaired physicians program (IPP) available; of them, 48 percent were run by the state medical societies, 28 percent by the state boards, 20 percent jointly run, and 8 percent run by a private contractor.
70. Alcohol and drug abuse was generally accepted by the 1960s as a medical issue (Conrad and Schneider 1992).
71. *JAMA* (1974: 524).
72. Pelton (1995), reprinted in the program materials in CAC (1998a). They had a 78 percent success rate measured as two years of sobriety, but 7 percent of those reentered the program. Since 1992 they no longer accept sexual offenders. In a long letter to the members of the Sunset Review Committee (November 17, 1997, included in CAC 1998b), Julianne Fellmouth of the Center for Public Interest Law at the University of San Diego argued that this program did not adequately protect the public.
73. Ruecki (1997: 1–2).
74. Goetz (1995: 131).
75. Dobson, Resnick, and Ulwelling (1994).
76. Oregon Board of Medical Examiners Report (1993: 1).
77. Oregon Board of Medical Examiners Report (1993: 2).
78. Allen (1995).
79. Hankes (1995).
80. See the Ad Hoc Committee on Physician Impairment's (1994) report on chemical dependency.
81. Hankes (1995); Vanderberry (1995).
82. Thompson (1975: 44).
83. Vanderberry (1995).
84. See the Ad Hoc Committee on Physician Impairment's (1995) report on sexual boundary issues.
85. This was from a speech at the FSMB 1966 meeting by the chair of the California Medical Association (Anderson 1966: 400).
86. Illinois State Medical Society (1972: 498).
87. Bohler (1973: 419–420).
88. Curry (1976: 4).
89. North Carolina Medical Board (1968); Alexander (1988: 281).

Chapter 4 — The State, the Media, and the Shaping of Public Opinion

1. The requirements for foreign-trained physicians still vary considerably among states, particularly in the number of years required for a U.S.-approved residency.

2. Shaw (1957: 67–68).
3. Wolfe (1993: 233).
4. Schudson (1995: 217).
5. For an excellent analysis and description of the transition to discipline that emphasizes the importance of court cases in the process, see Ameringer (1999).
6. The Council on Licensure, Enforcement, and Regulation surveyed sunset legislation (CLEAR 1986) published a guide for legislatures on how to conduct sunset reviews (Carpenter 1987). But while its list in 1988 showed that thirty-one states still had sunset regulations, by 1997 only twenty-four states had retained them. Kearney (1990) shows that state legislatures that repealed sunset legislation have few staff members, pay low salaries, and have low professionalism.
7. Although public members were a topic of discussion at the conference, no public members spoke.
8. Shimberg (1980: 31, 119, 120, 183).
9. National Center for the Study of Professions (1979: 5).
10. National Center for the Study of Professions (1980b: 2).
11. National Center for the Study of Professions (1980a: 1).
12. Kearney (1990).
13. Abel (2011) found that in California the press was also a major contributor to changes in regulating lawyers.
14. Schudson (1995: 25).
15. An investigation by the *Cleveland Plain Dealer* in April 1985 lead to direct changes in the Medical Practice Act, according to the associate director of education of the Ohio Medical Association (Porter 1986: 678).
16. Until the American Association of Retired Persons (AARP) in the late 1980s started to fund the CAC, few public-interest groups were interested in boards.
17. When Brown (2009) interviewed both reporters and legislators, both sides acknowledged the importance of the media in legislative decision making. Most legislators were skeptical of polls, and they read media sources with their own filters combined with interest group and public opinion in making decisions. Despite the democratic hope for the role of the press as a means to teach or communicate issues to the public, a frame for understanding them, and galvanizing it to action, neither Brown nor I have much evidence that it does so.
18. While this may not be "public journalism" as described by Fischer (2009), as it is not directly in dialogue with the broader public, it calls attention to an issue that most of the public are unaware, thus bringing the topic into the public discourse.
19. About twenty articles in the series "Dangerous Doctors: A Medical Dilemma" appeared in the *Miami Herald* between February 27, 1979, and December 2, 1979. The main investigation, by Carl Hiaasen, Patrick Malone, and Gene Miller, was laid out in eight articles: "Why Bad Doctors Get Away with It," "Bad Doctors Shielded by 'Silence,'" "'Conspiracy of Silence' Hides Bad MDs," "Watchdogs—Too Slow, Too Protective," "Discipline by Board Is Lenient," "Courts Put Chastised Doctors Back in Business," "Few Feel Osteopathic Board's Punishment Clout," and "Sickly Discipline System Faces 'Knife'" (Hiaasen, Malone, and Miller 1979a–1979h).
20. National Center for the Study of Professions (1981a: 4).
21. Hiaasen, Malone, and Miller (1979a).
22. Miller (1979).
23. Hiaasen, Malone, and Miller (1979e).
24. *Miami Herald* (1979).

25. Hiaasen (1979).
26. Malone (1979).
27. Astler (1974: 177).
28. Palmer (1975: 42–43).
29. Thompson (1975: 44).
30. The Florida Medical Association (FMA) president wrote that the FMA counsel did a "masterful job of amendment drafting and wording revisions at key moments. . . [The] FMA role in this highly politicized society is not only a professional group but as a key factor in trying to keep alive a free society in our state and nation" (Hodes 1979: 667).
31. Tash and Harper (1982a, 1982b).
32. Feinstein (1983: 44, 46).
33. Feinstein (1985: 801, 804).
34. In 1985 they added two additional public members.
35. National Center for the Study of Professions (1981b: 4).
36. National Center for the Study of Professions (1981b: 4).
37. An article in 1986, written by Michael Young, a lawyer for the TMA, gave the board a glowing report.
38. Sorelle (1992a). The series of articles (Sorelle 1992a–1992d) were forwarded to me on May 4, 1998, by Ruth Sorelle, and all appeared under her byline.
39. Sorelle (1992a).
40. Sorelle (1992a).
41. Sorelle (1992b).
42. Sorelle (1992c).
43. Sorelle (1992d).
44. Knox and McGrory (1992: 1, 28).
45. Bass (1993: 26).
46. Kong (1994a). The entire 1994–1995 *Globe* series was by Dolores Kong.
47. Kong (1994b).
48. Kong (1995a).
49. Kong (1995c).
50. Kong (1995b, 1995d).
51. Fleming (1997: 6–16).
52. Wielawski (1986b). The *Providence Journal* series is in Wielawski (1986a–1986b).
53. Wielawski (1986a).
54. Wielawski (1986c, 1986d).
55. Funk and Wielawski (1986).
56. Starkman (1986).
57. This series was authored by David Parrish and Jodie Snyder and appeared in the *Arizona Republic*, online edition. One article was entitled "No One Is Protecting the Public from Bad Medicine" (Parrish, Snyder, and Konig 2000). Another was entitled "Repeat Offenders Keep Working" (Parrish and Snyder 2000).
58. Only in about two-thirds of the states in the 1990s were doctors required to do continuing education for licensure. Most of the medical specialty boards require continuing education credits to maintain certification, but not all doctors are board certified.
59. Wolfe (2003).
60. Public Citizen found local medical society resistance in 1974 when it started to publish a consumer directory of questionable doctors (Ameringer 1999: 3, 61).

61. Allen (2002). When Dr. Wolfe gave a presentation at the 2005 FMSB meetings, the Maryland board members again objected to his ranking system.

62. Robeznieks (2002). *American Medical News* (amednews.com) is a news website oriented toward physicians.

63. American Association of Retired Persons (1993). Board administrators, who sometimes felt that they were not actively included in FSMB, formed this group in 1984, and the CAC worked with them.

64. There have been some efforts to remedy this situation by educating the public. For example, the People's Medical Society, founded in 1983, had a website and newsletter to inform the public about medical errors and how to prevent them. Charles Inlander, coauthor of *Medicine on Trial* (Inlander, Levin, and Weiner 1988), argues that consumers have the right to be informed when something goes wrong, as he says he stated in his testimony before the National Summit on Medical Errors and Patient Safety Research: "We ask this esteemed panel to carefully consider the consumer in your deliberations and recommend a course of action that not only reduces medical errors, but also recognizes that consumers have the right to be fully informed about the outcome of all medical procedures" (Quality Interagency Coordination Task Force 2000).

65. The Federation, in public, expresses the opinion that the boards need to be tough disciplinarians and has spoken out regularly about how rigorous the boards have become. In a *JAMA* article, James Winn, MD, executive vice president of FSMB, is quoted as saying, "We are trying to make individual boards more efficient and responsive to complaints. . . . It's our feeling that more can be done in the area of medical discipline. . . . Are we satisfied? . . . No we're not" (Marwick 1994: 1723).

66. Kusserow, Handley, and Yessian (1987: 820–824); CAC (1992a: 4).

67. AMA Board of Trustees (1986).

68. Several letters appeared in *JAMA* (1986).

69. The OIG appears to be the only federal agency interested in medical boards after the 1970s. Its reports include "Medical Licensure and Discipline: An Overview" (OIG 1986), "State Medical Boards and Discipline" (OIG 1990), "State Medical Boards and Quality of Care Cases" (OIG 1993), and "Managed Care Organization Nonreporting to the National Practitioner Data Bank" (OIG 2001). Mark Yessian, who was a primary author of these reports, also wrote a number of articles under his own name (1994a, 1994b). He is also a board member of CAC and has spoken at Federation annual meetings.

70. Title IV of the Health Care Quality Improvement Act of 1986 gave legal protection to those referring cases to the state medical boards, and most states increased their mandatory reporting laws (1986–1990). The PROs' predecessors were peer standards review organizations (PSRO), funded by the federal government to decide if Medicare services were necessary, met professional standards, and were provided in appropriate settings. In 1982 they became PROs; however, PRO strategies have been largely educational (Yessian and Greenleaf 1997).

71. OIG (2001).

72. An executive order of October 26, 1987, and February 16, 1990, pushed the Public Health Service to support state efforts (OIG 1993).

73. From October 1, 1988, to December 31, 1989, only 349 sanction notices were issued by PROs (OIG 1990: 28).

74. The Health Care Finance Administration (HCFA), the AMA, and ASPE(Assistant Secretary for Planning and Evaluation, HHS) opposed the proposal that the PROs share information on doctors with the state medical boards.

75. Nevertheless, Sidney Wolfe, writing for Public Citizen in the OIG report "State Medical Boards and Medical Discipline" (OIG 1990), wanted to expand the reforms by increasing public membership of the boards to 30 percent, weakening the relationship between medical societies and the boards, disseminating more information, strengthening board authority, opening the National Practitioner Data Bank to the public, encouraging complaints, keeping courts in check, hiring more investigators, and increasing board funding.

76. This OIG report (1990) explains that licensing fees were not getting to the boards and that the U.S. Department of Health and Human Services (HHS) 1987 Task Force on Medical Liability and Malpractice had urged states to fund boards so that they could perform their disciplinary function—but had little effect.

77. CAC (1992b, 1993, 1994).

78. Not including Hawaii, Tennessee, and Pennsylvania Osteopathic.

79. In Nevada and Oklahoma the allopathic (MD) organizations must, but not the osteopathic (DO) facilities (Federation Exchange 1999–2000: 38–39).

80. In Oklahoma MDs must report, but not DOs (FSMB 1999–2000: 38–39).

81. In Oklahoma, Nevada, and Vermont, the MD professional associations must report, but not the DO organizations (FSMB 1999–2000: 38–39).

82. North Carolina Medical Board (1999: 179).

83. In Arizona, the DO board does, but not the MD; in California, Oklahoma, West Virginia, and New Mexico, the MD does, but not the DO board. Six states did not answer (FSMB 1999–2000: 38–39).

84. Reilly (1995). In the appellate case Arnett v. Dal Cielo, 36 Cal. App. 4th 639 (1995), it was decided that the boards could see the hospital peer review records in the California Supreme Court (Arnett v. Dal Cielo, 96 Daily Journal D.A.R. 12129, decided October 3, 1996); and see CAC (1997: 2).

85. FSMB (1998).

86. AMA and FSMB (1995).

87. Pear (2001).

88. Ameringer (1999: 86–92) provides an analysis of a case in which the New Jersey board sought information on the doctors in an impairment program (New Jersey v. Jacobs, Civil No 93–3670, slip op. at 3–4 [D.N.J. Oct. 5, 1993]), which affected many states.

89. Schware v. Board of Bar Examiners, 353 U.S. 232 (1957).

90. Albert (2002).

91. These data are from FSMB (2006). Note that in four states the MD and DO boards have different standards.

92. These observations are further supported by Grad and Marti's (1979) research on medical boards in the 1970s. They saw little improvement during the period 1960–1977.

93. This quote was in the 1992 audit of state health-regulatory boards (Division of State Audit, Suite 1600, James Polk State Office Building, Nashville, TN) and was quoted in the *CAC News* (CAC 1992c). The Health Occupations Council requested a study (Chesney, n.d.) of public members in Michigan that showed that many public members actively participated in their boards, though some appeared more active than others (Chesney 1984).

94. I obtained the years from the state statutes.

95. Spaulding (1997: 83).

96. Public members are not representative of the population of the states, and many who use deliberative democracy as a model might argue that public members

constitute an elite group. Some states try for geographic, gender, and racial diversity, but from my observations, most are older, wealthier, and better educated than the average.

97. Each year the CAC meetings became more organized with speakers and specific periods for discussion and with less time for telling stories and trying to figure out how other boards work. The first meetings provided many opportunities to learn how the other boards functioned.

98. Fawcett, Lurie, and Wolfe (2002).

99. The data banks make it more difficult for doctors to move undetected across state lines as the states can query the data banks before granting them a license. The Federation started a data bank in 1985 when only three out of fifty-four allopathic and one in nine osteopathic boards submitted data. After 1985, states rapidly began to submit their actions. The National Practitioner Data Bank (NPDB), legislated and funded by Congress in 1986 by the HCQIA, was not ready until 1990. The Department of Health and Human Services, the Health Resources and Service Administration, and the Bureau of Health Professions had data by 1990. The NPDB required reporting of all malpractice cases, disciplinary decisions by boards, and hospital and HMO's adverse actions.

100. Todd (1993: 226–230).

101. Wyden (1993: 224–225).

102. Wolfe (1993: 231–235).

103. Paxton (1993: 236–239). Anne Paxton was the editor of *Public Member*.

104. This does not include what sessions are open to the public as there is no source for obtaining this information.

105. All data are from the FSMB (1999–2000, including tables), and my indicator was developed with the following information: (1) educational/information programs (table 48), 6 points total: 3 points for public programs, 2 points for licensees programs, 1 point for medical students, 1 point for residents; (2) information release to citizens (table 35), 3 points total: 1 point for the nature of disciplinary actions, 1 point for current investigations, 1 point for current charges; (3) organizations release information to the following organizations (table 34), 5 points total: 1 point PRO, 1 point law enforcement, 1 point other licensing jurisdictions, 1 point hospitals, 1 point state hospital associations; (4) formal sharing with PRO (table 33), 1 point total: 1 point formal information sharing; (5) public record and sharing with other boards (table 32), 8 points total: 1 point includes complaints shared before investigation; 1 point investigation information before decision shared, 1 point informal actions for public record status and another for shared, 1 point for license applications denials for public records and another for shared, 1 point for examinations irregularity for public record and another for shared, N/A (not available) counted as zero; (6) newsletter (table 18), 2 points total: 1 point for newsletter, 1 point for providing state officials and media with newsletter access; (7) annual report (table 17), 4 points total: 1 point for annual report available to public, 1 point for identification of disciplinary actions, 1 point for ranked list type of discipline actions, 1 point for number of licensees impaired. The average score was 14.33, and the range was from 6 (not very transparent) to 26 (making their work transparent).

106. Shimberg and Greene (1982) use five models to describe differences and report that in 1969 the Council of State governments could identify only sixteen states that had a central agency involved (this was for all licensing boards, but not necessarily just licensing for physicians), but by 1980, twenty-nine states had a central agency involved.

107. I developed this indicator to further understand the relationship of the boards to the state. I weighed self-definition heavily but added other aspects of board organization to understand the variation in independence from the state (FSMB 1999–2000, including tables): (1) self-definition (table 1): 4 points autonomy, 3 semiautonomous, 2 subordinate, 1 advisory; (2) source of nomination medical members (table 3), 2 points medical association specific, 1 point for any medical organization or individual; (3) staff board relationship to the board (table 6), 1 point each of board authority to employ, direct activities, set compensation, evaluate performance, fire: 4–5 authorities = 3 points, 2–3 authorities = 2 points, 1–0 authorities = 1 point; (4) finances (table 13), 3 points board receives all money from licensure fees, 2 points if the board is required to give back some of the fees, 1 if the board gives all money to the general state funds and receives only a portion back; (5) set fees (table 14), 2 points if board sets fees, 1 point if others do so; (6) source of legal counsel (table 10), 3 points for board/private, 2 points for board attorney and attorney general, 1 point for attorney general). The range is 6 to 17. For state embedded boards, the state actors make at least some of the decisions and boards have few hiring and firing rights. Where state boards have separate MD and DO boards, most are organized similarly (FSMB 1999–2000).

108. In at least nineteen states the state medical society runs the impaired physician program (FSMB 1995). In FSMB (1999–2000), table 12 ("Special Programs Operated by the Board"), it appears that the medical societies run the impaired physicians committees in even more states, but the FSMB did not specifically ask, so the self-reported number is approximate and refers to the medical societies.

109. Wilson (1978: 567).

110. Andre (1980: 176).

111. Hood (1986: 226).

112. Marr (1986: 227–228).

113. Baum (1988).

114. Michigan Act 368 of 1978 was amended in 1993 (333.17021) to include ten physicians, one physician assistant, and eight public members after April 1, 1994.

115. Mettler (1971: 843).

116. Riggs (1979: 109).

117. Malta (1985: 287–288).

118. Lewis (1993: 147–148).

119. Carroll (1979: 400–401).

120. Bechamps (1987: 18, 20, 21).

121. Adams (2003).

122. Greene (2001).

123. Berman (1976: 42, 44, 45).

124. Coller (1976: 38).

125. Carden (1988: 206–210).

126. CAC (2002a).

127. CAC (2002a).

128. CAC (2002b).

129. Allen (2002).

130. FSMB (1999–2000).

131. Pew (1995a, 1995b). In December 1996, the CAC held a conference, "Continuing Professional Competence: Can We Assure It?," that included speakers from the Federation and the American Board of Medical Specialties in Washington, DC. The CAC also produced a report, "Maintaining and Improving Health Professional Competence," in 2004.

132. "Licensure and Regulation of Health Care Professionals" is a position paper of the FSMB (1997b).
133. A 1994 FSMB resolution called for a national license limited to telemedicine but failed (Pew 1995b: vii, ix, 5).
134. As the report was being written, licensing boards were beginning to post disciplinary actions on their websites; however, not much information about the individual cases was available (Pew 1995b: ix).
135. Pew (1995b: ix).
136. Winn (1995: 14).
137. Later in the "President's Message," Dr. James West discussed another break with the AMA on issues of pain management, where the AMA "proposed policies that may take away the state licensure agency's ability to discipline physicians when that physician claims to be treating chronic pain syndrome" (West 2008: 37).
138. Cain (2003: 23–34); Kohn et al. (2000).
139. Despite earlier efforts to defeat prior board changes, the president of the medical association was quoted as saying that "the Texas Medical Association has gone to bat for the Board of Examiners in previous sessions to get more funding" (Robeznieks 2002).
140. Several editorials in favor of assessing continued competency appeared in the *Federation Bulletin* by FSMB chairs (including Lankford [2007, 2008] and McCord [2007]).
141. For a discussion of the examination, see Scoles (2002).
142. Croasdale (2003, 2004).
143. This newsletter article is reprinted in the *Journal of Medical Licensure and Discipline* (2008) from the online version of the *Medical Board of California Newsletter*, published by the Medical Board of California.

Chapter 5 — Rhetorics of Law, Medicine, and Public Interest Shape Board Work

1. Compliance with the trend toward public members may be more symbolic than substantive, but research shows that even symbolic compliance can make a difference in the ways boards do their work (Suchman and Edelman 1996: 920–921). But research on public participation is pessimistic. For example, Barger and Hadden (1984) found that almost half of the board members saw their role as no different from that of the professional members and saw their effectiveness purely in terms of having participated in the discussion. Other researchers, who have focused on the participation of public members on Health Planning Councils, have found that public members do not seem to affect outcomes for a number of reasons, one of them being that administrators have the most influence and suggest that staff tend to use clarification and complementing to subvert the influence of public members. Some who have focused on medical boards argue that public members are intimidated or co-opted by the professional members or that their roles are unclear (Brownlea 1987; Checkoway 1981b, 1982; Chesney 1984; Dolan and Urban 1983; Graddy 1991; Hanson 1980; Klein 1973; Klein and Lewis 1976; Law and Hansen 2010; Miller 1988; Morone 1984; Paap and Hanson 1982; Schultz 1983; Svorny 1992, 1997). Yedidia (1980), for example, discusses the differences between lay and professional knowledge of health care and delivery that could influence the lack of public participation. But Graddy and Nichol (1990) found an increased proportion of public members associated with taking more serious disciplinary actions. There are so

many organizational, statutory, and interactional variations that it is difficult to measure percentage or numbers of public members and disciplinary outcomes.

2. Smith (1994: 81). As a result of a campaign by George Bernard Shaw and a publicized case, the first public member in England was appointed in May 23, 1926 (Smith 1994: 80).

3. Majoribanks, Delvecchio Good, Lawthers, and Peterson's (1996) research shows that medical competence in daily practice has been effectively challenged by law in the malpractice arena.

4. Based on this argument, Cohen's (1997) criterion of people being free from constraints for deliberative democracy to be legitimate is not met. However, while discursive domains may be weaker in other situations, people bring with them different tools in all settings and are rarely free from any constraints. Heimer (1999) and Heimer and Staffen (1998) show how the institutions of medicine, law, and the family conflict over decisions in neonatal care with each institution constraining the actors' choices.

5. Elster (1998).

6. Some research (Montgomery 1990, 1992) shows that physicians do change their perspectives when they become administrators, though Freidson (1986) argues that physician-administrators do not think differently than practicing physicians.

7. Where the public's lack of expertise becomes important is in deciding exactly what the nurses should and should not be permitted to do.

8. Although a debate exists between social scientists who see the profession as unified (Goode 1957; Larson 1977; Parsons 1964) and those, particularly the symbolic interactionists, who see many fragmentations (Bucher and Strauss 1961; Hughes 1994), here I am talking about a general consistency, but many divisions clearly occur.

9. The New York Public Interest Group Inc. (NYPIRG) trained public members on different types of boards; according to the National Center for the Study of Professions (1980c: 6–7), "We do not know how these public members were selected or what their experience is. They have no visible impact."

10. Research found that about 4 percent of New York hospital patients suffered complications from treatment that extended hospital stays or resulted in disability or death. One percent of admissions involved negligence (Leape 1994).

11. Hunter (1991: 50–55), a professor of English, followed doctors in a hospital and analyzed the narrative structures physicians use, for example, doctor's rounds, which include the nature of the request for care, the history of illness, the past medical history, the present social situation, a review of symptoms, the results of the physical exam, the test results, and nonfindings.

12. Hunter (1991: 70).

13. See Bucher and Stelling (1969); Rosenthal (1995). Hunter (1991: 37) argues that most physicians have a low tolerance for uncertainty and express opinions as strong beliefs.

14. Mizrahi (1984).

15. Gawande (2002: 56) also describes how he learned to do procedures on patients after watching, which did not work well the first few times he tried it, and patients may have suffered (2002: 33–34).

16. Bosk (1979).

17. Hunter (1991: 10); and see Bosk (1979) and Hunter (1991: 32–34).

18. For example, the California Medical Association formed a subsidiary, the Institute for Medical Quality, to provide consultations to individual physicians and hospitals

to maintain quality care; the results are confidential and educational and are not part of a disciplinary proceeding. Institute for Medical Quality (n.d.).

19. Orlander and Fincke (2003: 656–658).

20. Gawande (2002: 59–61).

21. In states where there are significant penalties for failure to report to the NPDB, more adverse actions are reported (Scheutzow 1999).

22. As the authors of the Center for Peer Review Justice website have stated, they want the peer review to be a legal process as they feel that they were poorly treated by their own experiences by peer review committees: "We are dedicated to the exposure, conviction, and sanction of any and all doctors, and affiliated hospitals . . . who would use peer review as a weapon to unfairly destroy other professionals" (Center for Peer Review Justice, n.d.).

23. Using FSMB data on disciplinary actions from 1999–2003 and 2004–2008, I tried to identify the percent of actions that would require knowledge of medicine, estimating a rate of about 11 percent between 1999 and 2003 and a rate of about 12 percent between 2004 and 2008. Other disciplinary actions involved sex and moral breaches (11 percent), criminal actions (11–12 percent), medical records (4–5 percent), prescribing (5–7 percent), impairment (9–7 percent), among others. As each state reports using its own categories, it is difficult to figure out what many of the actions are, for as there are almost one hundred categories. These numbers are approximate.

24. Collins and Evans (2006).

25. Epstein (2007) demonstrated that AIDS activists were important in contributing to medical knowledge. Here I note Fischer's (2009) objection to Collins and Evans (2006) view that appears to separate science and sociopolitical reasoning. One only has to see the eruption of protests in November 2009 over suggested changes in the frequency of mammogram use to see that even careful "nonpolitical" analysis involves some ethical choices (Kolata 2009: 4).

26. Some argue that juries are truly unable to make reasonable malpractice decisions.

27. Rosenthal (1995).

28. *Texas Medicine* (1973: 112).

29. Rockwell (1993: 42–44).

30. Sirianni (2009: 9). Sirianni argues that "consumers" are people to manipulate and persuade but that they do not have a role as stakeholders (59).

31. National Center for the Study of Professions (1980d: 6).

32. As quoted in CAC (1995: 1).

33. Yessian (1994a: 12).

34. Common in this debate is a confusion of the rights and duties of board members with their skills and perspectives. The former should be the same for all members, the latter are not. Yedidia (1980), for example, discusses differences in lay and professional knowledge of health and health care.

35. Bosk (1979: 46).

36. Andrews (2002: 71).

37. Yessian (1994b: 193).

38. Ad Hoc Committee on Physician Impairment (1995: 209).

39. Ad Hoc Committee on Physician Impairment (1995: 208–209).

40. This estimate is based on FSMB data, which the Federation calculated for me.

41. State employees are sometimes subject to state politics. One director told me that he could not get the attorney general to prosecute cases because he was running for office and wanted physician support. Other directors have been fired at least in part

because of Wolfe's rankings and a local exposé. One lost his job when he tangled with the medical society.

42. National Center for the Study of Professions (1981d: 4).

43. Andrew and Sauer (1996: 229). Both authors were board members, one a public member (Andrew) and the other a medical member (Sauer).

44. Swidey (2004) describes the case.

45. Schumacher (1999: 57).

46. Freidson's research shows most are unaware of others' problems (1975).

Chapter 6 — Medical and Legal Discourses in Investigatory Committees

1. The emphasis of discipline remains moral character, which appears to reflect a different trajectory than what Imber (2008) argues is the replacement of character by knowledge and skills, which has driven the wedge between doctors and patients. Bosk (1979) explains that this emphasis is deeply embedded in the account of "good-faith effort," to which the reactions of senior staff are much more significant, although technical errors are more prevalent.

2. Pellegrino (1994: 224, 227).

3. Shaw (1957: 105).

4. McIntyre and Crausman (2008). While the Centers for Medicare and Medicaid Services no longer pay for wrong-patient or wrong-sited surgeries (as of January 2009), problems continue, particularly when protocols are not followed (O'Reilly 2010).

5. Studies of international law have had to try to understand a variety of levels of legalization. Abbott et al. (2000) have developed three dimensions to examine the degree of legalization: obligation (the degree to which one is bound by law), precision (the degree of specificity of the laws), and delegation (which third party makes decisions and which parties are bound to their decisions). They do not see a bright line between legal and nonlegal. Here, too, the situation among the boards varies along a continuum. All physicians are required to follow state laws, yet the degree of specificity of those laws varies. Some have much more specific rules than others, yet many are just "standards" that require local medical experts to define, particularly with regard to negligence and incompetence. The dispute-settlement mechanisms are the boards; decisions are binding, but appealable to courts.

6. All of the dialogues used here are composites based on my many conversations with board members and staff across the country. The issues are those that board members told me about, some of which I also experienced. I heard similar stories from public and medical board members and staff across the country. The issues that came up most often I use here to discuss what some board members considered pivotal and what some public members experience when they attempt to be active board members. Sometimes public members said that they felt comfortable that they understood cases well enough to make reasonable assessments, but other times they did not. I tried to encourage them to think about the situations in which they felt they could make reasonable decisions and when they could not. We did not talk about the specifics of potentially problematic actions of doctors; we talked about how the cases were discussed and how members participated. Public members said they sometimes did not know whether a reasonable decision was made, particularly in cases that involved diagnoses and treatments. Sometimes they became angry at what they saw happening. Others saw no problems with the ways decisions were made. Boards have more than one way of discussing cases depending on who is

there, and they often evolve with new staff and members. Consequently, this analysis does not reflect a particular board or boards. To ensure the adequacy of my examples, I gave them to several people involved in board work to read and presented the two major discourses from the perspective getting the most out of public members at an FSMB annual meeting held April 22–24, 2010, in Chicago, Illinois.

7. Mansbridge (1983, 2003).

8. Some research on alternative dispute resolution (ADR) sees it as less formal and more adaptive to local situations. Although it may not be binding, it is often formal in the sense of elaborate rules, making it formal for the less powerful. Alternative dispute resolution, while it may be adaptive to the local environment, is consequential when one group has power over the other, particularly in business organizations where workers tend to be disadvantaged by ADR (Abel 1982; Edelman and Suchman 1997). The investigatory committee is formally organized by medical or legal discourse, and its outcome is consequential. It isn't peer review.

9. I am not making an argument opposing reason and emotion (Frankfurt School) as I see emotion as Mead does—alerting us to suffering and opening opportunities to ask whether the public is being protected (Shalin 1992).

10. Hafferty and Light (1995); Montgomery (1990, 1992).

11. In one state the board could define overcharging as misconduct and spent energy on cases of physicians who charged insurance companies for separate procedures that, the medical members argued, were really aspects of a single procedure (unbundling).

12. Marks (2004: 25–31). This approach could be characterized as "restorative" justice, as both sides are able to express their viewpoints informally and the perpetrator can acknowledge harm without consequences. The aim is to reduce future harm (Hudson 2005). Very few in this program appear before the board a second time.

13. Gawande (2002: 88–108).

14. No available data exists to compare how boards handle cases or the number of confidential or private actions they take.

15. See Hunter (1991) for a description of doctors' stories.

16. For example, one state reported that more than 50 percent of the physicians called in for interviews were for inappropriate prescribing and substance abuse (Newton and Stratas 1994: 23–34).

17. Hunter (1991: 10, 15, 19; quotation is on 10).

18. The NBME announced on its website on August 25, 2011, that as of January 1, 2012, only six tries would be permitted. An applicant who failed a section six times would not be permitted to take the next section. The USMLE has been the national exam given since 1992 by the NBME and is required of all new licensees.

19. Fischer (2009) argues that policy experts can play a facilitating role in deliberations, but here they are both facilitator (expert evaluation) and full debater in an uneven debate that gives them much more power. They get to control the information, debate, and vote.

20. Some lawyers gain the interactional competency described by Collins and Evans (2006, 2007), and they can discuss many details of what happened in negligence and incompetence cases. In hearings, many of the prosecutors seemed to have learned a significant amount about particular practices and could talk intelligently about complex medical cases and ask good questions. Nevertheless, the physicians' questions of the witnesses often filled in important details.

21. According to many deliberative democracy theorists, "rational" discourse without expression of emotions is a requirement (Benhabib 1996; Cohen 1998; Schumpeter

1976). But the situation is more complicated as emotions are often felt, as my experiences, described in Chapter 1, illustrate in addition to the emotions experienced by the staff and board members described above. The rehashing of cases over and over is also an expression of the emotions felt by board members when they have made a difficult decision. I would find it difficult to argue that emotions never color interactions or decisions or that it is negative that they do. Minimally it signals that something important is happening, and in the view of Nussbaum (2001) emotions are a source of awareness, critical judgment, and understanding. Emotions can have a positive impact on deliberations (Fischer 2009).

22. Williams and Williams (2008).

Chapter 7 — Hearing and Sanction Deliberations

1. Schmacher (2000: 103).
2. Shaw (1957: 74).
3. See Dickinson (2005: 6–13) for an analysis of the differences between preponderance of evidence and clear and convincing evidence.
4. In many states an ALJ may hear a case, but the board may change the findings of fact and the conclusions of law and decide the sanction. In a Federation survey, in fifty-four of sixty-six boards, all or part of the hearing is in front of the full board, and in forty-one boards at least part or some of the hearing is in front of a panel or special standing committee. Forty-nine used a hearing officer for some part of the process, but nine boards hold all hearings in front of the full board without a hearing officer. Three states hold the entire hearing in front of an ALJ without board member involvement (FSMB 1999–2000).
5. Some ALJs play an active role in the decision-making process and argue with panels as they wrestle with the opinion. The ALJs are supposed to write opinions as stated by the panel, but some interject themselves in the decision with their opinions.
6. On one occasion, during a hearing with the talk of the respondent having guns in his office, the panel became sufficiently frightened to ask for a security guard. In another case, the defense lawyer shouted at the panel and accused the ALJ of rigging the case against his client. Despite being instructed to sit down, he refused to. The panel and the ALJ were very upset. I got a stomachache. The lawyer was replaced.
7. I can't prove this point as either a sociologist or as a public member. I do know my notes are not always perfect; I do not have total recall. Thus, I assume that the establishment of "fact" and what was said at the hearing is not perfectly matched. Both as a sociologist and as a public member, I believe that my notes and memories adequately reflect what went on during the hearings, but I would have more confidence if I had had a transcript.
8. Pellegrino (1994).
9. According to stories repeated by board physicians, even a lesser sanction such as suspension or censure can lead to HMO suspension. I was unable to document any cases, but it is what many board members say when arguing about a sanction.
10. Federation data shows that a significant percentage of all physicians sanctioned have licenses in more than one state.
11. While Black (1984) argues that, in hearings where punishment is the goal, the focus is on the actions and, in hearings where rehabilitation is the goal, the focus is on the actor, here each is the focus of different participants and ends debated.
12. Mizrahi (1984).
13. Gutmann and Thompson (2004: 44).
14. Dewey (1954: 51).

Chapter 8 — Democratic Deliberation and the Public Interest

1. This is also the expression that Abel (2011) uses to describe the self-regulation of lawyers.
2. Freidson (1990, 2001).
3. Saks (1995).
4. Arrow (1963).
5. Smith, discussed in Dingwall and Fenn (1987).
6. Freidson (1990: 441).
7. Freidson (1990, 2001) suggests, following Collins (1979: 171), that groups create social closure as associational or consciousness communities, excluding all without correct credentials.
8. Freidson (2001: 217).
9. Freidson (2001); as well as Halpern and Anspach (1993).
10. Freidson (1975).
11. Ben-David (1963) and Parsons (1964: 70) argue that altruism bound only the doctor-patient relationship.
12. Freidson (2001: 217).
13. Freidson (2001: 202).
14. Mead (1962: 254–256).
15. Freidson (2001: 181).
16. Freidson (2001: 122–123).
17. See Freidson (2001: chapter 9).
18. Saks (1995) makes a strong effort to construct a way of deciding what is in the public interest. I do not try to do so. I am trying to set up a system that provides better debate and arrives at the public interest.
19. Abbott (1988) points to the jurisdictional claims among professions over work as the source of the growth of those who win—here we saw the conflicts over medical and legal claims of social control processes. It is partially this competition that permits public members sufficient resources to evaluate fully what was going on.
20. Bosk (1979: 168).
21. See Jacobs's (1977) analysis of Stateville Prison.
22. See Bohman and Rehg (1997); Dewey (1954); Gutmann and Thompson (2004); Habermas (1996); Mead (1962); Pateman (1970, 1985); Young (1997a, 1997b).
23. Dewey (1954: 213); Mead (1899: 369).
24. See Bohman and Rehg (1997); Bourdieu (1977); Elster (1998); Gutmann and Thompson (2004); Habermas (1996); Pateman (1970; 1985).
25. Pateman (1970).
26. See Elster (1998).
27. Gargarella (1998); also see Elster (1998).
28. In South Carolina the physicians are elected by region.
29. Pateman (1970: 64).
30. Nicolas Rose points toward a possible mechanism for avoiding some of the problems of the isolation of communities. Citizenship, beyond community membership, may come from membership in multiple communities: "zones of identity—lifestyle sectors, neighbourhoods, ethnic groups—some private, some corporate, some quasi-public." However, he argues that multiple memberships are not cumulative (Rose 1999: 178).
31. Young (1997a, 1997b).
32. Knight and Johnson (1997).

33. Pateman (1985).
34. Fischer (2009); Sirianni (2009).
35. Parsons's (1954) model is the best example of altruism and self-regulation while Berlant (1975), Freidson (1975), and Larson (1977) view medicine as grasping for power and thus should not be permitted to self-regulate. Research on numbers of disciplinary actions, flawed because of the many variations in boards, show that increased finances are consequential for disciplining more physicians, but the same research also shows that boards that work independently from the state also discipline a higher percentage of physicians. State oversight did not increase discipline (Law and Hansen 2010).
36. Early critiques of self-regulation as an undue market restriction include Benham (1980) and Pfeffer (1974), but some saw the need for self-regulation but with an improved process (Wolfson, Trebilcock, and Tuohy 1980).
37. Horowitz (2001); Mead (1962); Shalin (1986, 1988).
38. Mead (1962: 167–168).
39. Ferguson (2007).
40. Skocpol (2002).
41. This is recommendation is the opposite of what has been proposed by new governance scholars, who argue in favor of devolution today, and it is the opposite of the direction much regulation of industry has taken recently (Ayres and Braithwaite 1994).

Conclusion

1. Medical regulation combined one aspect of much regulation at the end of the nineteenth century—the belief that "science" could inform regulatory decisions objectively but without a cumbersome bureaucracy. According to Imber (2008), this same science model helped to diminish our trust in physicians.
2. Beginning in the 1970s, "evidence-based medicine" was intended to standardize the practice of medicine by providing practice standards and guidelines, or "best practices." Yet according to Hafferty (2003: 143–144), less than 50 percent of diagnosis and treatment procedures is "backed by hard scientific evidence in the 21st Century."
3. The European Union is working to make its nations' systems of regulation of medicine similar to each other to facilitate possible intercountry mobility.
4. Baker (2005) argues that large malpractice settlements and the likelihood of being sued are myths, but that has not deterred doctors from focusing on the cases that they know about or have heard of and worrying about their chances of being sued (Marjoribanks et al. 1996; Gawande 2002).
5. Hafferty (2003).

References

Abbott, A. 1988. *The System of Professions: An Essay on the Division of Expert Labor.* Chicago: University of Chicago Press.

———. 1999. "Ecologies Liées aux Environs du Système des Professions." Manuscript. Chicago: University of Chicago, Department of Sociology.

Abbott, K., R. Keohane, A. Moravesik, A.-M. Slaughter, and D. Snidal. 2000. "The Concept of Legalization." *International Organization* 54: 401–419.

Abel, R. 1982. *The Politics of Informal Justice.* New York: Academic Press.

———. 2011. *Lawyers on Trial.* New York: Oxford University Press.

Adams, D. 2003. "Virginia Law on Doctor Discipline Casts Wider Net." *American Medical News*, April 11. amednews.com (accessed April 14, 2003).

Ad Hoc Committee on Physician Impairment. 1994. "Report." *Federation Bulletin* 81(4): 229–242.

———. 1995. "Report on Sexual Boundary Issues." *Federation Bulletin* 82(4): 208–225.

Akers, R. 1968. "The Professional Association and the Legal Regulation of Practice." *Law and Society Review* 2: 463–482.

Albert, T. 2002. "Arizona Court Overturns Decision of Medical Board." *American Medical News*, October 7. amednews.com (accessed March 7, 2003).

Alexander, E. 1988. "The Board of Medical Examiners Explained." *North Carolina Medical Journal* 49: 281–282.

Allen, A. 1995. "Missouri Physicians' Health Foundation Impaired Physicians Program." *Federation Bulletin* 82: 141–145.

Allen, G. 1967. *William James.* New York: Viking.

Allen, T. 2002. "A New Approach to Medical Errors and Medical Discipline." *Maryland Psychiatrist* 28(2): 9–10.

Allsop, J. 2002. "Regulation and the Medical Profession." In *Regulating the Health Professions*, ed. Judith Allsop and Mike Saks, 79–93. London: Sage.

Allsop, J., and L .Mulcahy. 1996. *Regulating Medical Work.* Bristol, PA.: Open University Press.

Ameringer, C. 1999. *State Medical Boards and the Politics of Public Protection.* Baltimore: Johns Hopkins University Press.

AMA and FSMB. 1995. "Report of the American Medical Association and the Federation of State Medical Boards: Ethics and Quality of Care." *Federation Bulletin* 82(2): 90–93.

AMA Board of Trustees. 1986. "Report: AMA Initiative on Quality of Medical Care and Professional Self-Regulation." *JAMA* 256(8): 1036–1037.

AARP. 1993. "Survey of Public Members on Selected State Licensing Boards." Washington, DC: AARP and CAC.

Anderson, C.C. 1966. "California State Board and State Medical Associations." *Arizona Medicine* 23(5): 399–401.

Andre, H. M. 1980. "Medical Profession Burdened by Restrictions." *Michigan Medicine* 79: 176.

Andrew, G., and H. Sauer. 1996. "Do Boards of Medicine Really Matter?" *Federation Bulletin* 83: 228–236.

Andrews, L. 2002. "Public Members: The Voice of the Public." *Journal of Medical Licensure and Discipline* 88: 70–75.

Aronson, S., N. Deary, and M. Hamolsky. 1996. "The Licensed Physicians of Rhode Island in the Year 1895." *Medicine and Health/Rhode Island* 79(2): 60–67.

Arrow, K. J. 1963. "Uncertainty and the Welfare Economics of Medical Care." *American Economic Review* 111: 941–973.

Astler, V. B. 1974. "Probe of State Licensing Boards." *Journal of the Florida Medical Association* 61: 176–178.

Atiyah, P. S. 1979. *The Rise and Fall of Freedom of Contract.* Oxford: Oxford University Press.

Atkinson, P. 1995. *Medical Talk and Medical Work.* London: Sage.

Ayres, I., and J. Braithwaite. 1992. *Responsive Regulation.* New York: Oxford University Press.

Baggott, R. 2002. "Regulatory Politics, Health Professionals, and the Public Interest." In *Regulating the Health Professions*, ed. Judith Allsop and Mike Saks, 31–47. London: Sage.

Baker, S. L. 1984. "Physician Licensure Laws in the United States, 1865–1915." *Journal of the History of Medicine* 39: 173–197.

Baker, T. 2005. *The Medical Malpractice Myth.* Chicago: University of Chicago Press.

Barger, D., and S. Hadden. 1984. "Placing Citizen Members on Professional Licensing Boards." *Journal of Consumer Affairs* 18: 160–170.

Barnard, F. 1972. "The Germ Theory of Disease and Its Relations to Hygiene." In *Medical America in the Nineteenth Century*, ed. G. Brieger, 278–292. Baltimore: Johns Hopkins University Press.

Bass, A. 1993. "First Non-physician to Head Medical Board." *Boston Globe*, March 11.

Baum, J. K. 1988. "We Must Take an Active Role in Providing Quality Care." *Michigan Medicine* 87: 260.

Bechamps, G. J. 1987. "Innovation and Cooperation Enhance Policing Mechanism." *Virginia Medicine* 114: 18–21.

Becker, H. S., B. Geer, E. C. Hughes, and A. Strauss. 1961. *Boys in White.* Chicago: University of Chicago Press.

Bellin, L. E., F. Kavaler, and A. Schwartz. 1972. "Phase One of Consumer Participation in Policies of 22 Voluntary Hospitals in New York City." *American Journal of Public Health* 62: 1370–1378.

Ben-David, J. 1963. "Professions in the Class System of Present Day Societies." *Current Sociology* 12: 247–298.

Benhabib, S. 1996. "Toward a Deliberative Model of Democratic Legitimacy." In *Democracy and Difference: Contesting the Boundaries of the Political*, ed. S Benhabib, 67–94. Princeton, NJ: Princeton University Press.

Benham, L. 1980. "The Demand for Occupational Licensure." In *Occupational Licensure and Regulation*, ed. S. Rottenberg, 13–25. Washington, DC: American Enterprise Institute.

Benham, L., and A. Benham. 1975. "Regulating through the Professions: A Perspective on Information Control." *Journal of Law and Economics* 18: 421–447.

Berlant, J. 1975. *Profession and Monopoly.* Berkeley: University of California Press.

Berman, J. I. 1976. "Legal Mechanisms for Dealing with the Disabled Physician in Maryland: Partnership between the Medical Society and the State Commission on Medical Discipline." *Maryland State Medical Journal* 25: 41–45.

Bigelow, H. 1972. "Insensibility during Surgical Operations Produced by Inhalation." In *Medical America in the Nineteenth Century*, ed. G. Brieger, 169–175. Baltimore: Johns Hopkins University Press.

Black, D. 1984. *Toward a General Theory of Social Control*, vol. 1. New York: Academic Press.

Blendon, R., and J. M. Benson. 2001. "Americans' Views on Health Policy: A Fifty Year Historical Perspective." *Health Affairs* 20: 33–46.

Bohler, C. E. 1973. "Presidents Letter: Mechanism for Medical Discipline." *Journal of the Medical Association of Georgia* 62: 419–420.

Bohman, J. 1997. "Deliberative Democracy and Effective Common Reason: Capabilities, Resources, and Opportunities." In *Deliberative Democracy*, ed. J. Bohman and W. Rehg, 321–348. Cambridge, MA: MIT Press.

Bohman, J., and W. Rehg, eds. 1997. *Deliberative Democracy: Essays on Reason and Politics*. Cambridge, MA: MIT Press.

Bosk, C. 1979. *Forgive and Remember*. Chicago: University of Chicago Press.

Bourdieu, P. 1977. *Outline of a Theory of Practice*. Cambridge: Cambridge University Press.

Brieger, G., ed. 1972. *Medical America in the Nineteenth Century*. Baltimore: Johns Hopkins University Press.

Brint, S. 1994. *In an Age of Experts*. Princeton, NJ: Princeton University Press.

———. 2005. "Guide for the Perplexed: On Michael Burawoy's "Public Sociology." *American Sociologist* 36: 46–65.

Brown, E. K. 2009. "Public Opinion and Policy Making." Ph.D. dissertation, UMI 3348184. State University of New York at Albany. Microform.

Brownlea, A. 1987. "Participation: Myths, Realities and Prognosis." *Social Science and Medicine* 25: 605–614.

Bucher, R., and J. Stelling 1969. "Characteristics of Professional Organizations." *Journal of Health and Social Behavior* 10: 3–15.

Bucher, R., and A. Strauss. 1961. "Professions in Process." *American Journal of Sociology* 66: 325–334.

Budd, J. 1978. "Bierring Lecture." *Federation Bulletin* 65: 131–138.

Burawoy, M. 2005. "For Public Sociology." *American Sociological Review* 70: 4–28.

Burnham, J. 1972. "Medical Specialists and Movements toward Social Control in the Progressive Era." In *Building the Organizational Society*, ed. J. Israel, 19–30. New York: Free Press.

CAC. 1992a. "Information Exchange between Peer Review Organizations and Medical Licensing Boards." Washington, DC: CAC.

———. 1992b. "A Resource Guide for Seeking to Limit Judicial Stays of Board Disciplinary Orders." Washington, DC: CAC.

———. 1992c. "State of Tennessee Issues of Performance Audit of Health-Related Boards." *CAC News* 4(2): 7–8.

———. 1993. "Allocation of Decision-Making Authority between Board Members and Staff." Fall. Washington DC: CAC.

———. 1994. "Use of Alternative Dispute Resolution by Health Professions Licensing Boards." November. Washington DC: CAC.

———. 1995. "Public Representation on Health Care Regulatory, Governing and Oversight Bodies." In *Workshop Proceedings (May 1994)*. Washington, DC: CAC.

———. 1997. "Hospital Reporting to State Regulators." Washington, DC: CAC.

———. 1998a. Program materials. In *Forum on the Regulatory Management of Chemically Dependent Health Care Practitioners*, ed. CAC. Key Bridge Marriott, Arlington, VA, March 5–6. Washington, DC: CAC.

———. 1998b. "Briefing Book." In *Forum on the Regulatory Management of Chemically Dependent Health Care Practitioners*, ed. CAC. Key Bridge Marriott, Arlington, VA, March 5–6. Washington, DC: CAC.

———. 2002a. "State Official Says Professional Association Too Close to Disciplinary Process." *News and Views* 13(3): 3–4.

———. 2002b. "Maryland Legislators Propose Changes in Medical Board Operations." *News and Views* 14(1): 22–23.

———. 2004. "Monitoring and Improving Health Professional Competence." April. Washington, DC: CAC.

Cain, F. 2003. "Maintenance of Licensure and the Medical Profession." *Journal of Medical Licensing and Discipline* 89: 23–34.

Caldwell, L. 1923. "Early Legislation Regulating the Practice of Medicine." *Illinois Law Review* 18: 225–244.

Caplow, T. 1954. *The Sociology of Work.* Minneapolis: University of Minnesota Press.

Carden, E. 1988. "Whither the Impaired Physician? The Politics of Impairment." *Maryland Medical Journal* 37: 206–210.

Carpenter, E. 1987. "The Heath Occupations under Review: An Update on State Sunrise Activities, 1985–87." Report for the National Clearinghouse on Licensure Enforcement and Regulation and the Council of State Governments. Ann Arbor, MI: Gini Associates. Mimeographed.

Carroll, G. 1979. "Disciplining the Errant Physician: In Virginia, Investigations Show an Increase." *Virginia Medicine* 106: 400–401.

Carr-Saunders, A. P., and P. A. Wilson. 1933. *The Professions.* Oxford: Oxford University Press.

Cassedy, J. 1991. *Medicine in America.* Baltimore: Johns Hopkins University Press.

Center for Peer Reviewed Justice. N.d. www.peerreview.org (accessed March 23, 2004).

Chafetz, M., and G. Chafetz. 1994. *Obsession: The Bizarre Relationship between a Prominent Harvard Psychiatrist and Her Suicidal Patient.* New York: Random House.

Chase-Dunn, C. 2005. "Global Public Social Science." *American Sociologist* 36: 121–132.

Checkoway, B. 1981a. "Citizens and Health Care in Perspective: An Introduction." In *Citizens and Health Care: Participation and Planning for Social Change*, ed. B. Checkoway, 1–17. New York: Pergamon Press.

———. 1981b. "Innovative Citizen Participation in Health Planning Agencies." In *Citizens and Health Care: Participation and Planning for Social Change*, ed. B. Checkoway, 118–138. New York: Pergamon Press.

———. 1982. "Public Participation in Health Planning Agencies: Promise and Practice." *Journal of Health, Policy, Politics and Law* 7: 723–733.

Chesney, J. N.d. "A Report on the Role and Effectiveness of Public Members on Licensing Boards." Report presented to the governor and legislature by the Health Occupations Council. Ann Arbor: University of Michigan, School of Public Health.

———. 1984. "Citizen Participation on Regulatory Boards." *Journal of Health Policy, Politics, and Law* 9: 125–135.

Cirn, J. 1980. "The Birth Throes of the Wisconsin Medical Practice Act: The Physicians versus the Newspaper Editors." *Wisconsin Medical Journal* 79: 12–14.

CLEAR. 1986. "Survey of Sunset Legislation." Lexington KY: mimeograph.

Cohen, H. S. 1973. "Professional Licensure, Organizational Behavior, and the Public Interest." *Milbank Memorial Fund Quarterly* 51: 232–247.

———. 1975. "Regulatory Politics and American Medicine." *American Behavioral Scientist* 19: 122–135.

———. 1980. "On Professional Power and Conflict of Interest: State Licensing Boards on Trial." *Journal of Health Politics, Policy, and Law* 5: 291–308.

Cohen, H., and L. Miike. 1973. "Developments in Health Manpower Licensure." HEW. Washington, DC: U.S. Government Printing Office.

———. 1974. "Toward a More Responsive System of Professional Licensure." *International Journal of Health Services* 4:265–272.

Cohen, J. 1997. "Procedure and Substance in Deliberative Democracy." In *Deliberative Democracy*, ed. J. Bohman and W. Rehg, 407–438. Cambridge, MA: MIT Press.

———. 1998. "Democracy and Liberty." In *Deliberative Democracy*, ed. J. Elster, 185–231. Cambridge: Cambridge University Press.

Coller, J. 1976. "The Commission on Medical Discipline of Maryland." *Maryland State Medical Journal* 25: 35–39.

Collins, H., and R. Evans. 2006. "The Third Wave of Science Studies." In *The Philosophy of Expertise*, ed. E. Selinger and R. Crease, 39–110. New York: Columbia University Press.

———. 2007. *Rethinking Expertise*. Chicago: University of Chicago Press.

Collins, R. 1979. *The Credential Society*. New York: Academic Press.

Conrad, P., and J. Schneider. 1992. *Deviance and Medicalization*. Philadelphia: Temple University Press.

Consumer Reports. 2011. "Medical Errors," poll. Appendix: Questionnaire, February 8. NRC no. 2010.130. Yonkers, NY: Consumer Reports National Research Center.

Creighton, L. 1976. *Pretenders to the Throne*. Lexington, MA: D. C. Health.

Croasdale, M. 2003. "AMA against NBME's Clinical Skills Test." *American Medical News*, July 7, amednews.com (accessed May 9, 2012).

———. 2004. "AMA Takes Aim at Skills Exam." *American Medical News*, July 5, amednews.com (accessed May 9, 2012).

Curry, L. 1976. "What It Is Like to Be Involved as a Peer in the Medical Practice Act." *Journal of the Medical Association of Georgia* 65: 3–4.

Dary, D. 2008. *Frontier Medicine*. New York: Knopf.

Derber, C., W. Schwartz, and Y. Magrass. 1990. *Power in the Highest Degree*. New York: Oxford University Press.

Derbyshire, R. 1965. "What Should the Profession Do about the Incompetent Physician?" *JAMA* 194: 119–122.

———. 1966. "The Objectives and Achievements of State Medical Board Licensure Examinations." *JAMA* 198(7): 758–759.

———. 1969. *Medical Licensure and Discipline in the United States*. Baltimore: Johns Hopkins University Press.

———. 1973. "How Effective Is Medical Self-Regulation?" *Law and Human Behavior* 7(3): 193–202.

———. 1974. "Medical Ethics and Discipline." *JAMA* 228: 59–62.

———. 1976a. "Medical Licensure and Professional Discipline." Editorial. *JAMA* 85: 384–385.

———. 1976b. "Comments on a Proposal for 'Credentialing' Health Manpower." *Federation Bulletin* 63(9): 291–298.

Dewey, J. 1954. *The Public and Its Problems*. Athens: Ohio University Press. Originally published 1927.

Dickinson, J. 2005. "The Disparity in State-based Quality of Care Disciplinary Standards." *Journal of Medical Licensure and Discipline* 94: 6–13.

Dingwall, R. 1976. "Accomplishing Profession." *Sociological Review* 24: 331–349.

Dingwall, R., and P. Fenn. 1987. "A Respectable Profession?" *International Review of Law and Economics* 7: 51–64.

Dingwall, R., and P. Hobson-West. 2006. "Litigation and the Threat to Medicine." In *Challenging Medicine*, ed. D. Kelleher, J. Gabe, and G. Williams, 46–64. London: Routledge.

Dobson, D., M. Resnick, and J. Ulwelling. 1994. "Remediation versus Discipline in Oregon." *Federation Bulletin* 81(1): 14–18.

Dolan, A., and N. Urban. 1983. "The Determinants of the Effectiveness of Medical Disciplinary Boards, 1960–77." *Law and Human Behavior* 7: 203–217.

Duffy, John. 1993. *From Humors to Medical Science: A History of American Medicine*. Chicago: University of Illinois Press.

Durkheim, E. 1992. *Professional Ethics and Civic Morals*. New York: Rutledge.

Eaton, D. 1972. "The Essential Conditions of Good Sanitary Administration." In *Medical America in the Nineteenth Century*, ed. G. Brieger, 293–300. Baltimore: Johns Hopkins University Press.

Edelman, L., and M. Suchman. 1997. "Legal Environments and Organizational Governance." *Annual Review of Sociology* 23: 479–515.

Edmondson, F. 1971. "Competence and Quality of Medical Care" *JAMA* 216(11): 1855.

Eisner, M. 1993. *Regulatory Politics in Transition*. Baltimore: Johns Hopkins University Press.

Elshtain, J. 1995. *Democracy on Trial*. New York: Basic Books.

Elster, J. 1998. "Introduction." In *Deliberative Democracy*, ed. J. Elster, 1–18. Cambridge: Cambridge University Press.

Epstein, S. 2007. *Inclusion*. Chicago: University of Chicago Press.

Erichsen, J. 1972. "Impressions of American Surgery." In *Medical America in the Nineteenth Century*, ed. G. Brieger, 182–189. Baltimore: Johns Hopkins University Press.

Etzioni, A. 1996. *The New Golden Rule*. New York: Basic.

Evans, R. 1980. "Professionals and the Production of Function." In *Licensing and Regulation,* ed. S. Rottenberg, 225–264. Washington, DC: American Enterprise Institute.

Fawcett, J., P. Lurie, and S. Wolfe. 2002. "Survey of Doctor Disciplinary Information on Web Sites." Health Research Group report no. 1615, April 9. Washington, DC: Public Citizen.

Federal Interagency Council on Citizen Participation. 1977. "At Square One: Proceedings of the Conference on Citizen Participation in Government Decision Making," December 1976. Washington, DC: Federal Interagency Council on Citizen Participation.

Feinstein, R. J. 1983. "My Experiences as a Member of the Florida State Board of Medical Examiners." *Journal of the Florida Medical Association* 70: 43–46.

———. 1985. "The Ethics of Professional Regulation." *New England Journal of Medicine* 312: 801–804.

Ferguson, R. 2007. *The Trial in American Life*. Chicago: University of Chicago Press.

Fischer, F. 2009. *Democracy and Expertise*. New York: Oxford University Press.

Fitz, R. H. 1894. "The Rise and Fall of the Licensed Physician in Massachusetts, 1781–1860." *JAMA*: 22(23): 877–883.

Fleming, A. 1997. "Massachusetts Physician Profiles." *Federation Bulletin* 84: 6–16.

Flexner, A. 1910. *Medical Education in the United States and Canada: A Report to the Carnegie Foundation for the Advancement of Teaching*. Bulletin no. 4. New York: Carnegie Foundation.

Flint, A. 1866. *A Treatise on the Principles and Practice of Medicine*. Philadelphia: H. C. Lea.

———. 1972. "Conservative Medicine." In *Medical America*, ed. G. Brieger, 134–142. Baltimore: Johns Hopkins University Press.

Forgotson, E. H., and J. Cook. 1967. "Innovations and Experiments in Uses of Health Manpower—The Effect of Licensure Laws." *Law and Contemporary Problems* 32: 731–750.

Forgotson, E. H., and R. Roemer 1968. "Government Licensure and Voluntary Standards for Health Personnel and Facilities." *Medical Care* 6: 345–354.

Forgotson, E. H., R. Roemer, and R. W. Newman. 1967a. "Licensure of Physicians." *Washington University Law Quarterly*, 1976(3): 249–331.

———. 1967b. "Licensure of Physicians." Report of the National Advisory Commission on Health Manpower. Washington, DC: U.S. Government Printing Office.

Foucault, M. 1973. *The Birth of the Clinic.* New York: Random House.

Freidson, E. 1970a. *The Profession of Medicine.* New York: Harper & Row.

———. 1970b. *Professional Dominance.* Chicago: Aldine.

———. 1973. "Prepaid Healthcare and the New "Demanding" Patient." *Milbank Memorial Fund Quarterly* 51: 473–488.

———. 1975. *Doctoring Together: A Study of Professional Social Control.* Chicago: University of Chicago Press.

———. 1984. "The Changing Nature of Professional Control." *Annual Review of Sociology* 10: 1–20.

———. 1986. *Professional Powers: A Study of the Institutionalization of Formal Knowledge.* Chicago: University of Chicago Press.

———. 1990. "The Centrality of Professionalism to Health Care." *Jurimetrics* 30: 431–445.

———. 2001. *Professionalism, the Third Logic.* Chicago: University of Chicago Press.

Friedman, L. 1965. "Freedom of Contract and Occupational Licensing: 1890–1900: A Legal and Social Study." *California Law Review* 53: 487–534.

Friedman, M. 1962. *Capitalism and Freedom.* Chicago: University of Chicago Press.

FSMB. 1921. "Report: Rhode Island." *Federation Bulletin* (January): 5.

———. 1993. "Survey of State Medical Boards Regarding Impaired Physician Programs." Euless TX: FSMB.

———. 1995. "Federation Exchange." Euless, TX: FSMB.

———. 1997a. "Awareness and Attitudes about State Medical Boards." Survey, photocopied. Euless, TX: FSMB.

———. 1997b. "Licensure and Regulation of Health Care Professionals." *Federation Bulletin* 84: 94–110.

———. 1998. "Report of the Special Committee on Evaluation of Quality of Care and Maintenance of Competence." *Federation Bulletin* 85: 35–43.

———. 1999–2000. "Federation Exchange." Euless, TX: FSMB.

———. 2006. "Trends in Physician Regulation." Euless TX: FSMB.

Funk, M., and I. Wielawski. 1986. "Medical Review Board Decides to Revoke Dr. Balasco's License." *Providence Journal*, February 27.

Gallagher, W. T. 1995. "Ideologies of Professionalism and the Politics of Self-Regulation in the California State Bar." Unpublished manuscript. San Francisco: Townsend and Townsend Khourie and Crew.

Gambetta, D. 1998. "'Claro!' An Essay on Discursive Machismo." In *Deliberative Democracy*, ed. J. Elster, 19–43. Cambridge: Cambridge University Press.

Gardner, H. 1980. "Bierring Lecture." *Federation Bulletin* 67: 361–363.

Gargarella, R. 1998. "Full Representation, Deliberation and Impartiality." In *Deliberative Democracy*, ed. J. Elster, 260–280. Cambridge: Cambridge University Press.

Garland, D. 2001. *The Culture of Control.* Chicago: University of Chicago Press.

Gawande, A. 2002. *Complications.* New York: Holt.

———. 2007. *Better.* New York: Holt.

Gilb, C. 1966. *Hidden Hierarchies.* New York: Harpers.

Goetz, R. 1995. "The Florida Practitioners Program." *Federation Bulletin* 82: 131–133.

Goode, 1957. "Community within a Community: The Professions." *American Sociological Review* 22: 194–200.

Goodwin, J., J. Jasper, and F. Poletta. 2001. *Passionate Politics: Emotional and Social Movements.* Chicago: University of Chicago Press.

Grad, F., and N. Marti. 1979. *Physicians' Licensure and Discipline.* Dobbs Ferry, NY: Oceana Publications.

Graddy, E. 1991. "Interest Groups or the Public Interest—Why Do We Regulate Health Occupations?" *Journal of Health Politics, Policy, and Law* 16: 25–49.

Graddy, E., and M. B. Nichol. 1990. "Structural Reforms and Licensing Board Performance." *American Politics Quarterly* 18: 376–400.

Gray, J. F. *The policy of chartering colleges of medicine: being an introductory lecture to a course on the theory and practice of physic, delivered . . . November 5, 1832.* New York : H. Ludwig, printer, 1833.

Greene, J. 2001. "Physicians Win Big over Scope-of-Practice Issues." *American Medical News*, July 2. amednews.com (accessed August 3, 2002).

Gross, S. J. 1984. *Of Foxes and Hen Houses.* Westport, CT: Quorum Books.

Gunn, J. C. 1830. *Gunn's domestic medicine, or poor man's friend. Shewing the diseases of men, women and children, and expressly intended for the benefit of families. Containing a description of the medicinal roots and herbs, and how they are to be used in the cure of diseases . . .* 1st ed. Knoxville, TN: Printed by F. S. Heiskell, 1830.

Gutmann, A., and D. Thompson. 2004. *Why Deliberative Democracy?* Princeton, NJ: Princeton University Press.

Haber, S. 1991. *The Quest for Authority and Honor in the American Professions, 1750–1900.* Chicago: University of Chicago Press.

Habermas, J. 1996. *Between Facts and Norms: Contributions to a Discourse Theory of Law and Democracy.* Cambridge, MA: MIT Press.

Hafferty, F. 2003. "Review Symposium on Eliot Freidson's Professionalism." *Journal of Health Politics, Policy, and Law* 28: 133–158.

Hafferty, F., and D. Light 1995. "Professional Dynamics and the Changing Nature of Medical Work." *Journal of Health and Social Behavior* 35: 132–153.

Halpern, S., and R. Anspach. 1993. "The Study of Medical Institutions." *Work and Occupations* 20: 279–295.

Hankes, L. 1995. "Washington Physicians Health Program." *Federation Bulletin* 82: 158–163.

Hanson, B. 1980. "An Ethnography of Power Relations." *Research in the Sociology of Health Care* 1: 137–187.

Happel, T. J. 1901. "Enforcement of Medical Laws Dependent on an Organized Profession." *JAMA* 37: 1301–1303.

Haskell, T., ed. 1984. *The Authority of Experts.* Bloomington: Indiana University Press.

Haug, M. 1973. "Deprofessionalization: An Alternate Hypothesis for the Future." *Sociological Review Monograph* 20: 195–211.

———. 1980. "The Sociological Approach to Self-Regulation." In *Regulating the Professions*, ed. R. Blair and S. Rubin, 61–80. Lexington, MA: D. C. Heath.

Haug, M., and B. Lavin. 1981. "Practitioner or Patient: Who's in Charge?" *Journal of Health and Social Behavior* 22: 212–229.

———. 1983. *Consumerism in Medicine.* Beverly Hills, CA: Sage.

Heimer, C. 1999. "Competing Institutions: Law, Medicine, and Family in Neonatal Care." *Law and Society Review* 33: 17–66.

Heimer, C., and L. Staffen. 1998. *For the Sake of the Children*. Chicago: University of Chicago Press.

Held, D. 1996. *Models of Democracy*. Stanford, CA: Stanford University Press.

Hershey, N. 1969. "An Alternative to Mandatory Licensure of Health Professionals." *Hospital Progress* 50: 70–78.

HEW. 1971. "Report on Licensure and Related Health Personnel Credentialing." Washington, DC: U.S. Government Printing Office.

———. 1976. "A Proposal for Credentialing Health Manpower." Subcommittee on Health Manpower Credentialing of the Public Health Service Manpower Coordinating Committee. Washington, DC: U.S. Government Printing Office.

———. 1977. "Credentialing Health Manpower." Subcommittee on Health Manpower Credentialing of the Public Health Service Manpower Coordinating Committee. Washington, DC: U.S. Government Printing Office.

Hiaasen, C. 1979. "Professional Regulation Bill OKed." *Miami Herald*, May 4.

Hiaasen, C., P. Malone, and G. Miller. 1979a. "Why Bad Doctors Get Away with It." *Miami Herald*, February 25.

———. 1979b. "Bad Doctors Shielded by 'Silence.'" *Miami Herald*, February 26.

———. 1979c. "'Conspiracy of Silence' Hides Bad MDs." *Miami Herald*, February 27.

———. 1979d. "Watchdogs—Too Slow, Too Protective." *Miami Herald*, February 28.

———. 1979e. "Discipline by Board Is Lenient." *Miami Herald*, March 1.

———. 1979f. "Courts Put Chastised Doctors Back in Business." *Miami Herald*, March 2.

———. 1979g. "Few Feel Osteopathic Board's Punishment Clout." *Miami Herald*, March 3.

———. 1979h. "Sickly Discipline System Faces 'Knife.'" *Miami Herald*, March 4.

Hirschman, A. O. 1997. *The Passions and the Interests*. Princeton, NJ: Princeton University Press.

Hodes, R. 1979. "Keeping a Free Society Alive." *Journal of the Florida Medical Association* 66: 666–667.

Hoffman, C. 1973. "Half-Truths versus Wisdom: Bierring Lecture." *Federation Bulletin* 60(4): 114–126.

Hood, R. 1986. "Assuring Physician Competency in Michigan." *Michigan Medicine* 85: 224–226.

Horns, H. 1975. "Challenges to and Responses of the Federation of State Medical Boards." *Federation Bulletin* 62: 77–82.

Horowitz, R. 2001. "Inequalities, Democracy, and Fieldwork." *Symbolic Interaction* 24: 481–504.

———. 2009. "Public Membership on Medical Licensing Boards: An Integrated Public and Professional Project." In *Handbook of Public Sociology*, ed. V. Jeffries, 299–318. New York: Rowman & Littlefield.

Hudson, B. 2005. "The Culture of Control: Choosing the Future." In *Managing Modernity: Politics and the Culture of Control*, ed. M. Matravers, 49–75. New York: Routledge.

Hughes, E. C. 1958. *Men and Their Work*. New York: Free Press.

———. 1994. *On Work, Race, and the Sociological Imagination*. Chicago: University of Chicago Press.

Hunter, K. 1991. *Doctors' Stories*. Princeton, NJ: Princeton University Press.

Illich, I. 1976. *Medical Nemesis*. New York: Random House.

Illinois State Medical Society. 1972. "Recommendations on Health Care Licensure." *Illinois Medical Journal* 142(5): 497–504.

Imber, J. 2008. *Trusting Doctors*. Princeton, NJ: Princeton University Press.

Inlander, C., L. Levin, and E. Weiner. 1988. *Medicine on Trial*. New York: Prentice Hall.

Jacobs, J. 1977. *Stateville*. Chicago: University of Chicago Press.

JAMA. 1902a. "National Board of Medical Examiners." Editorial. 38–2: 108–109.

———. 1902b. "Medical Legislation." Editorial. 39–5: 317.

———. 1974. "Disabled Physicians Act." AMAGRAMS. 229(4): 524.

———. 1986. Letters. 390(1): 313–316.

Johnson, D., G. F. Dillon, and T. R. Henzel. 2000. "Post Licensure Assessment System." *Federation Bulletin* 88: 116–122.

Johnson, T. 1972. *Professions and Power*. London: Macmillan.

———. 1995. "Governmentality and Institutionalization of Expertise." In *Health Professions and the State in Europe*, ed. T. Johnson, G. Larkin, and M. Saks, 7–24. London: Routledge.

Jost, T., ed. 1997. *The Regulation of the Healthcare Professions*. Chicago: Health Administration Press.

Journal of Medical Licensure and Discipline. 2008. "Does National Licensure Make Sense?" 94(3): 37.

Judicial Council of the AMA. 1970. "Report." *JAMA* 213(4): 588.

Kearney, R. 1990. "Sunset: A Survey and Analysis of State Experience." Mimeographed. Columbia: University of South Carolina, Department of Government and International Studies.

Kelleher, D. 2006. "Self-Help Groups and Their Relationship to Medicine." In *Challenging Medicine*, ed. J. Gabe, D. Kelleher, and G. Williams, 104–121. London: Routledge.

Kelly, H. E. 1925. *Regulation of Physicians by Law: A Dissertation on Regulation by Law of the Occupation of Healing Diseases of Human Beings*. Chicago: American Medical Association.

Kennedy, J. F. 1963. "Special Message to the Congress on Protecting the Consumer Interest." In *Public Papers of the Presidents of the United States, 1962*, 235–238. Washington, DC: U.S. Government Printing Office.

Kinkel, R., and N. Josef. 1991. "Disciplining Doctors: How Medical Boards Are Dealing with Problem Physicians in the Midwest." *Research in the Sociology of Health Care* 9: 207–231.

Klein, R. 1973. *Complaints against Doctors: A Study in Professional Accountability*. London: Charles Knight.

Klein, R., and J. Lewis. 1976. *The Politics of Consumer Representation*. London: Centre for Studies in Social Policy.

Knight, J., and Johnson, J. 1997. "What Sort of Equality Does Deliberative Democracy Require?" In *Deliberative Democracy*, ed. W. Rehg and J. Bohman, 279–320. Cambridge, MA: MIT Press.

Knox, R., and B. McGrory. 1992. "Bean-Bayog Offers to Resign: Board Says No." *Boston Globe*, September 18.

Kohn, L. T., J. M. Corrigan, and M. S. Donaldson, eds. 2000. *To Err Is Human*. Washington, DC: National Academy Press, Institute of Medicine.

Kolata, Gina. 2009. "Get a Test. No Don't. Repeat." *New York Times*, November 22.

Kong, D. 1994a. "In Shift, Medical Groups Supports Disclosure." *Boston Globe*, November 18.

———. 1994b. "A Doctor's Past: Does the Public Have a Right to Know?" *Boston Globe*, November 28.

———. 1995a. "More Data on Doctors Is Urged at Hearing: Medical Board Called 'Stuporous.'" *Boston Globe*, February 3.

———. 1995b. "30 Hospitals Report Actions against Doctors." *Boston Globe*, April 20.

———. 1995c. "Public Has the Right to Files on Doctors, Panel Says." *Boston Globe*, May 3.

———. 1995d. "Survey: Fatalities Go Unreported" *Boston Globe*, July 30.

Kusserow, R., E. Handley, M. Yessian. 1987. "An Overview of State Medical Discipline." *JAMA* 257: 820–824.

Lankford, S. 2007. "Medical Boards a Key Element of Emerging Alliance for Physician Competence." *Federation Bulletin* 93: 3.

———. 2008. "Professionalism and Maintenance of Competency: Two Sides of the Same Coin." *Federation Bulletin* 94: 3.

Larson, M. S. 1977. *The Rise of Professionalism: A Sociological Analysis*. Berkeley: University of California Press.

———. 1984. "The Production of Expertise and the Constitution of Expert Power." In *The Authority of Experts*, ed. T. Haskell, 28–80. Bloomington: Indiana University Press.

Law, M., and Z. Hansen. 2010. Medical Licensing Board Characteristics and Physician Discipline." *Journal of Health Politics, Policy, and Law* 35(1): 63–93.

Leape, L. 1994. "Error in Medicine." *JAMA* 272: 1851–1857.

Lewis, S. 1993. "Both Ends of the Elephant." *Federation Bulletin* 80: 147–148.

Light, D. 1991. "Professionalism as a Countervailing Power." *Journal of Health Politics, Health Policy, and the Law* 16: 499–506.

Malone, P. 1979. "State Takes Over Policing of Doctors" *Miami Herald*, December 2.

Malta, F. J. 1985. "Medical License: Cherished Possession." *Journal of the Medical Society of New Jersey* 82: 287–288.

Mansbridge, J. 1983. *Beyond Adversary Democracy*. Chicago: University of Chicago Press.

———. 2003. "Practice-Thought-Practice." *Deepening Democracy*, ed. A. Fung and E. Wright, 175–199. New York: Verso.

Marjoribanks, T., M. J. Delvecchio Good, A. G. Lawthers, and L. M. Peterson. 1996. "Physicians' Discourses on Malpractice and the Meaning of Medical Malpractice." *Journal of Health and Social Behavior* 37: 163–178.

Marks, A. 2004. "Two-Call Case Resolution." *Journal of Medical Licensure and Discipline* 90: 25–31.

Marr, J. 1986. "Interview." *Michigan Medicine* 85: 227–230.

Marwick, C. 1994. "State Medical Boards Discipline More, Want Role in Health System Reform." *JAMA* 271(22): 1723–1724.

Maurizi, A. 1974. "Occupational Licensing and the Public Interest." *Journal of Political Economy* 82: 99–413.

McCleery, R. 1971. *One Life—One Physician: A Report to the Center for the Study of Responsive Law*. Washington, DC: Center for the Study of Responsive Law.

McCord, J. 2007. "A Shared Mission of Public Protection." *Journal of Medical Licensure and Discipline* 93: 3.

McCready, L., and B. Harris. 1995. "From Quackery to Quality Assurance: The First Twelve Decades of the Medical Board of California." Sacramento: Medical Board of California.

McIntyre, B., and R. Crausman. 2008. "A History of Wrong Site Surgery in Rhode Island." *Journal of Medical Licensure and Discipline* 94: 6–10.

McNamara, E. 1994. *Sex, Suicide, and the Harvard Psychiatrist*. New York: Pocket Books.

Mead, G. H. 1899. "The Working Hypothesis in Social Reform." *American Journal of Sociology* 5: 367–371.

————. 1962. *Mind, Self, and Society*. Chicago: University of Chicago Press. Originally published 1934.

Mechanic, D. 2006. *The Truth about Health Care*. New Brunswick, NJ: Rutgers University Press.

Medical Society of North Carolina. 1852. *Transactions*, 3: 96.

Memel, S. 1977. "A Note." *Federation Bulletin* 63: 157.

Merchant, F. 1970. "Challenges to Medical Licensing Board." *JAMA* 212(11): 1949–1951.

Mettler, F. A. 1971. "Is There an Equivalent in the House?" *Journal of the Medical Society of New Jersey* 68: 829–844.

Miami Herald. 1979. "Let the Medical-Examiner Board Use Scalpel on the Unethical." Editorial, October 21.

Millard, P. H. 1887. "The Propriety and Necessity of State Regulation of Medical Practice." *JAMA* 9: 491–493.

Millenson, M. 1997. *Demanding Medical Excellence*. Chicago: University of Chicago Press.

Miller, E. J. 1988. "Public Members on Professional Regulatory Boards: The Case of Lawyers in Wisconsin." *Administration and Society* 20: 369–390.

Miller, G. 1979. "Patient: He Forced Me to Have Sex," *Miami Herald*, February 25.

Millerson, G. 1964. *The Qualifying Associations*. London: Routledge.

Mizrahi, T. 1984. "Managing Medical Mistakes: Ideology, Insularity, and Accountability among Internists in Training." *Social Science and Medicine* 19: 135–146.

Montgomery, K. 1990. "A Prospective Look at the Specialty of Medical Management." *Work and Occupations* 17: 178–198.

————. 1992. "Professional Dominance and the Threat of Corporatization." In *Current Research in on Occupations and Professions*, ed. J. Levy, 221–240. Greenwich, CT: JAI Press.

Moran, M. 2002. "The Health Profession in International Perspective." In *Regulating the Health Professions*, ed. J. Allsop and M. Saks, 19–30. London: Sage.

————. 2004. "Governing Doctors in the British Regulatory State." In *Governing Medicine*, ed. A. Gray and S. Harrison, 27–36. Berkshire: Open University Press.

More, E. S. 1999. *Restoring the Balance: Women Physicians and the Profession of Medicine, 1850–1995*. Cambridge, MA: Harvard University Press.

Morone, J. A. 1984. "The Citizen Role in Health Politics: Democratic Wishes and Sensible Reforms." In *Health Politics and Policy*, ed. T. Litman and L. Robins, 243–57. New York: John Wiley.

Morrow, C. 1985. "The Medicalization of Professional Self-Governance: A Sociological Assessment." In *Social Control and the Medical Profession*, ed. J. Swazey and S. Scher, 163–183. Boston: Oelgeschlager, Gunn, & Hain.

Morton, J. 1975. "The Public on Boards?" *Federation Bulletin* 62(6): 184–185.

————. 1976. "Health Manpower Credentialing." Position paper. *Federation Bulletin* 63(11): 340–351.

————. 1980. "P Is for Public." *Federation Bulletin* 67: 146–147.

Morton, W. J. 1976. "Insuring Competence and Improving Discipline through the Medical Practice Act." *Journal of the Medical Association of Georgia* 65: 1–2.

National Center for the Study of Professions. 1979. "Common Cause on Sunset: 'A Powerful Concept.'" *ProForum* 1(9): 3, 5.

————. 1980a. "White House Challenges States to Reform Occupational Regulation." *ProForum* 2(8): 1.

————. 1980b. "Common Cause President: Sunset and Other Reforms Needed to Combat Special Interests." *ProForum* 2(8): 2.

————. 1980c. "New York Group Schedules Public Member Training Conference." *ProForum* 3(3): 6–7.

————. 1980d. "NCHCA Offers Guideline for the Selection of Public Members." *ProForum* 3(3): 6.

————. 1981a. "Florida Boards Cope with Publicity, Increases Discipline, and Toll-Free Complaint Line." *ProForum* 3(12): 4–5.

————. 1981b. "Medical Board Falls to Sunset Temporarily." *ProForum* 4(1): 4.

————. 1981c. "California Splits with Federation of State Medical Boards." *ProForum* 3(9): 2.

————. 1981d. "Regulating the Professions: Is There an Ideal Way?" *ProForum* 3(9): 1, 3, 4, 5.

Newton, L., and N. Stratas. 1994. "Review of Informal Interviews and Disciplinary Actions by the North Carolina Board of Medical Examiners." *Federation Bulletin* 81: 23–34.

North Carolina Medical Board. 1968. "Medical Licensure in North Carolina." *North Carolina Medical Journal* 29: 179–181.

————. 1999. "Professional Obligation to Report Incompetence, Impairment, and Unethical Conduct." *Federation Bulletin* 86: 46.

Nussbaum, M. 2001. *Upheavals of Thought: The Intelligence of Emotions.* Cambridge: Cambridge University Press.

————. 2004. *Hiding from Humanity: Disgust, Shame, and the Law.* Princeton, NJ: Princeton University Press.

OIG. 1986. "Medical Licensure and Discipline: An Overview." P-01–86–00064. Washington, DC: Health and Human Services.

————. 1990. "State Medical Boards and Medical Discipline." OEI-01–89–00560. Washington, DC: Health and Human Services.

————. 1993. "State Medical Boards and Quality of Care Cases." OEI-01–92–00050. Washington, DC: Health and Human Services.

————. 2001. "Managed Care Organization Nonreporting to the National Practitioner Data Bank." OEI-01–99–00690. Washington, DC: Health and Human Services.

Oldmixon, Mr. [J.]. 1741. *The British Empire in America: Containing the history of the discovery, settlement, progress and state of the British colonies on the continent and islands of America: Being an account of the country, soil, climate, product and trade of Newfoundland, New-England, New-Scotland, New-York, New-Jersey, Pensylvania, Maryland, Virginia, Carolina, Georgia, Hudson's-Bay.* 2nd ed., corrected and amended. 2 vols. London: Printed for J. Brotherton [and 9 others].

Oregon Board of Medical Examiners.1993. "Report." *Newsletter* (Spring): 1–2.

O'Reilly, K. 2010. "Wrong-Patient, Wrong-Site Procedures Persist despite Safety Protocol." *American Medical News*, November 1. amednews.com (accessed March 26, 2012).

Orlander, J. D., and B. G. Fincke. 2003. "Morbidity and Mortality Conference: A Survey of Academic Internal Medicine Departments." *Journal of General Internal Medicine* 18: 656–658.

Paap, W. R., and B. Hanson. 1982. "Unobtrusive Power: Interaction between Health Care Providers and Consumers at Council Meetings." *Urban Life* 10: 409–423.

Palmer, G. S. 1975. "Peer Discipline: We Have the Tools." *Journal of the Florida Medical Association* 62: 42–43.

Parrish, D., and J. Snyder. 2000. "Repeat Offenders Keep Working." *Arizona Republic*, August 21.

Parrish, D., J. Snyder, and R. Konig. 2000. "No One Is Protecting the Public from Bad Medicine." *Arizona Republic*, August 20.

Parsons, T. 1951. *The Social System*. New York: Free Press.

———. 1964. "The Professions and Social Structure." In *Essays in Sociological Theory*, ed. T. Parsons, 34–49. New York: Free Press.

———. 1970. "Definitions of Health and Illness." In *Social Structure and Personality*, ed. T. Parsons, 257–291. New York: Free Press.

Pateman, C. 1970. *Participation and Democratic Theory*. Cambridge: Cambridge University Press.

———. 1985. *The Problem of Political Obligation: A Critique of Liberal Theory*. Cambridge: Cambridge University Press.

Paxton, A. 1993. "The Tide against Secrecy." *Federation Bulletin* 80: 236–239.

Pear, R. 2001. "Inept Physicians Are Rarely Listed as Law Requires." *New York Times*, May 29.

Pellegrino, E. 1994. "Ethical Issues in Character Assessment and Medical Licensure." *Federation Bulletin* 81: 222–228.

Pelton, C. 1995. "The Medical Board's Diversion Program." January. Sacramento: Medical Board of California.

Pescosolido, B., S. Tuch, and J. Martin 2001. "The Profession of Medicine and the Public." *Journal of Health and Social Behavior* 42: 1–16.

Pew. 1995a. "Reforming Health Care Workforce Regulation: Policy Considerations for the 21st Century." Report of the Taskforce on Health Care Workforce Regulation. San Francisco: Pew Health Professions Commission.

———. 1995b. "Critical Challenges: Revitalizing the Health Professions for the Twenty-First Century." San Francisco: Pew Health Professions Commission.

Pfeffer, J. 1974. "Administrative Regulation and Licensing: Social Problem or Solution?" *Social Problems* 21: 468–479.

Porter, S. 1986. "The Ohio State Medical Board." *Ohio State Medical Journal* 82: 677–683.

Procter, I. M., and D. Long. 1959. *One Hundred Year History of the North Carolina State Board of Medical Examiners, 1859–1959*. Raleigh, NC: Edwards & Broughton.

Putnam, R. N. 2000. *Bowling Alone*. New York: Simon & Schuster.

Quality Interagency Coordination Task Force. 2000. Fact Sheet for the National Summit on Medical Errors and Patient Safety Research, September 11. Washington, DC. www.quic.gov/summit/summit.htm (accessed May 11, 2012).

Rayack, E. 1967. *Professional Power and American Medicine*. Cleveland: World Publishing.

Reilly, T. 1995. "Court Ruling on Peer Review Records." *Action Report, Medical Board of California* 55(October): 1.

Rhode Island Tribune. 1919. "Dr. Robbins Gets Five-Year Term." *Rhode Island Tribune*, October 18.

———. 1921. "Dr. A. O. Robbins in Court To-Day." *Rhode Island Tribune*, June 18.

Riddle, J. 1976. "Education and Medical Licensure." *JAMA* 236: 3041–3043.

Riggs, J. 1979. "Regulations, Licensure, Medical Discipline, and Self-Regulation of Physicians." *Journal of the Medical Society of New Jersey* 76: 109–113.

Robeznieks, A. 2002. "Analysis of States' Disciplinary Rates Raises Patient Safety Concerns." *American Medical News*, May 13. amednews.com (accessed November 25, 2002).

Rockwell, G. 1993. "The Role and Function of the Public Member." *Federation Bulletin* 80: 42–44.

Rodwin, M. 1994. "Patient Accountability and Quality of Care: Lessons from Medical Consumerism and Patient Rights, Women's Health, and Disability Rights Movements." *American Journal of Law and Medicine* 20:147–167.

Roemer, R. 1973. "Legal Systems Regulating Health Personnel." In *Politics and Law in Health Care Policy*, ed. J. McKinlay, 233–273. New York: Prodist.

Rose, N. 1999. *Powers of Freedom*. Cambridge: Cambridge University Press.

Rosenberg, C. E. 1979. "The Therapeutic Revolution: Medicine, Meaning, and Social Change in 19th Century America." In *The Therapeutic Revolution*, ed. M. J. Vogel and C. E. Rosenberg, 3–29. Philadelphia: University of Pennsylvania Press.

Rosenkrantz, B. G. 1974. "Cart before the Horse: Theory, Practice, and Professional Image in American Public Health, 1870–1920." *Journal of the History of Medicine* 29:55–73.

Rosenthal, M. 1995. *The Incompetent Doctor*. Buckingham, UK: Open University Press.

Rouse, M. 1968. "Bierring Lecture." *Federation Bulletin* 55: 75–77.

Rubin, L. B. 1969. "Maximum Feasible Participation: The Origins, Implications and Present Status." *Annals of the American Academy of Political and Social Science* 385(1): 14–29.

Ruecki, V. 1997. "Nevada State Board of Medical Examiners Diversion Program." *Newsletter of the Nevada State Board of Medical Examiners*.

Saks, M. 1995. *Professions and the Public Interest*. London: Routledge.

———. 2006. "The Alternatives to Medicine." In *Challenging Medicine*, ed. J. Gabe, D. Kelleher, and G. Williams, 84–103. London: Routledge.

Scheutzow, S. 1999. "State Medical Peer Review." *American Journal of Law and Medicine* 25: 7–60.

Schlesinger, M. 2002. "A Loss of Faith: The Sources of Reduced Political Legitimacy for the American Medical Profession." *Milbank Quarterly* 80: 185–235.

Schudson, M. 1995. *The Power of News*. Cambridge, MA: Harvard University Press.

———. 1998. *The Good Citizen*. Cambridge, MA: Harvard University Press.

Schultz, H. G. 1983. "Effects of Increased Citizen Membership on Occupational Licensing Boards in California." *Policy Studies Journal* 11: 504–516.

Schumacher, A. 1999. "President's Message." *Federation Bulletin* 86: 57.

———. 2000. "President's Message." *Federation Bulletin* 86: 103.

Schumpeter, J. 1976. *Capitalism, Democracy, and Liberalism*. London: Allen & Unwin.

Scoles, P. 2002. "An Evaluation of Clinical Skills in the United States Medical Licensing Examiners: A Report from the National Board of Medical Examiners." *Journal of Medical Licensing and Discipline* 88: 66–69.

Seguin, E. 1972. "Clinical Thermometry." In *Medical America in the Nineteenth Century*, ed. G. Brieger, 143–151. Baltimore: Johns Hopkins University Press.

Shadid, M. 1939. *A Doctor for the People*. New York: Vanguard Press.

Shalin, D. 1986. "Pragmatism and Social Interactionalism." *American Sociological Review* 51: 9–29.

———. 1988. "G. H. Mead, Socialism, and the Progressive Agenda." *American Journal of Sociology* 93: 913–951.

———. 1992. "Critical Theory and the Pragmatist Challenge." *American Journal of Sociology* 98: 237–280.

Shaw, G. B. 1957. *The Doctor's Dilemma*. London: Penguin. Originally published 1911.

Shimberg, B. 1980. "Occupational Licensing: A Public Perspective." Princeton, NJ: Educational Testing Services.

Shimberg, B., B. F. Esser, and D. H. Kruger. 1972. *Occupational Licensing: Practices and Policies*. A Report of the Educational Testing Service. Washington, DC: Public Affairs Press.

Shimberg, B., and K. Greene. 1982. "Improving Occupational Regulation: A Case Study in Federal-State Cooperation." U.S. Department of Labor Employment and Training Administration.

Shryock, R. 1966. *Medicine in America*. Baltimore: Johns Hopkins University Press.

———. 1967. *Medical Licensing in America, 1650–1965*. Baltimore: Johns Hopkins University Press.

Sirianni, C. 2009. *Investing in Democracy*. Washington, DC: Brookings Institution Press.

Skocpol, T. 2002. *Diminished Democracy: From Membership to Management in American Civic Life*. Norman: University of Oklahoma Press.

Smith, R. G. 1994. *Medical Discipline: The Professional Conduct Jurisdiction of the General Medical Council, 1858–1990*. Oxford: Clarendon Press.

Sorelle, R. 1992a. "Dangerous Practice, an Ailing System." *Houston Chronicle*, August 30.

———. 1992b. "Understaffing Mars Monitoring of Doctors on Probation." *Houston Chronicle*, August 31.

———. 1992c. "Critics of State Medical Board Take Aim at Loose Rules on Doctors." *Houston Chronicle*, September 1.

———. 1992d. "Medical Board Studies Vast Rule Changes—Push for Accountability." *Houston Chronicle*, October 10.

Southern Governors' Conference Resolution. 1976. "Health Manpower Licensure." *Federation Bulletin* 63(11): 350–351.

Spaulding, S. 1997. "President's Message." *Federation Bulletin* 84(2): 83–84.

Special Committee on Evaluation of Quality of Care and Maintenance of Competence. 1998. "Report." *Federation Bulletin* 85(1): 35–43.

Spencer, H. 2002. *Principles of Sociology*. New Brunswick, NJ: Transactions Publishers. Originally published 1898.

Stacey, M. 1992. *Regulating British Medicine: The General Medical Council*. Chichester, UK: Wiley.

Starkman, D. 1986. "Lawyer Blames Bad Doctors for Rising Insurance Costs." *Providence Journal*, February 22.

Starr, P. 1982. *The Social Transformation of American Medicine*. New York: Basic Books.

Stein, J. J. 1968. "Board of Medical Examiners, Recent Changes in Laws Relating to Practice in California." *California Medicine* 109: 53–58.

Stevens, R. 1998. *American Medicine and the Public Interest: A History of Public Interest*. Berkeley: University of California Press.

Stewart, F. C. 1972. "The Actual Condition of Medical Education in This Country." In *Medical America in the Nineteenth Century*, edited by G. Brieger, 62–74. Baltimore: Johns Hopkins University Press.

Stewart, J. B. 1999. *Blind Eye*. New York: Touchstone.

Stigler, A. 1971. "The Theory of Economic Regulation." *Bell Journal of Economic and Management Science* 2: 13–21.

Still, J. 1973. *Early Recollections and Life of Dr. James Still, 1812–1885*. New Brunswick, NJ: Rutgers University Press. Originally published 1877.

Suchman, M., and L. Edelman 1996. "Legal Rational Myths: The New Institutionalism and the Law and Society." *Law & Social Inquiry* 21: 903–941.

Svorny, S. 1992. "Should We Reconsider Licensing Physicians?" *Contemporary Policy Issues* 10: 31–38.

———. 1997. "State Medical Boards: Institutional Structure and Board Policies." *Federation Bulletin* 84: 111–119.

Swidey, N. 2004. "What Went Wrong?" *Boston Globe Magazine*, March 21.

Tash, P., and J. Harper. 1982a. "Delays, Light Penalties Mark Discipline of Professionals." *St. Petersburg Times*, January 31.

———. 1982b. "Regulation of Doctors Is Inconsistent." *St. Petersburg Times*, February 1.

Tennent, J. [1734]. *Every man his own doctor: or, The poor planter's physician: Prescribing, plain and easy means for persons to cure themselves of all, or most of the distempers, incident to this climate, and with very little charge, the medicines being chiefly of the growth and production of this country. Philadelphia: Reprinted and sold by B. Franklin.*

Texas Medicine. 1973. "Texas State Board of Medical Examiners—Effective, Quality Boardmanship." 69: 110–112.

Theobald, J. *Every man his own physician: being, a complete collection of efficacious and approved remedies, for every disease incident to the human body . . .* London: Printed and sold by W. Griffin, 1764.

Thompson, W. W. 1975. "Our Golden Opportunity." *Journal of the Florida Medical Association* 62: 44.

Tissot, [S. A. D.]. 1765. *Advice to the People in General, with Regard to their Health,* trans. J. Kirkpatrick, London: Printed for T. Becket and P. A. De Hondt.

Todd, J. 1993. "National Practitioner Data Bank: Worthy of Consumer Confidence?" *Journal of Medical Licensure and Discipline* 80: 226–230.

Vanderberry, R. 1995. "The North Carolina Physicians Health Program." *Journal of Medical Licensure and Discipline* 82:146–150.

Vevier, C. 1987. "The Flexner Report and Change in Medical Education." In *Flexner: 75 Years Later,* ed. C. Vevier, 1–11. Lanham, MD: University Press of America.

Vidmar, N. 1995. *Medical Malpractice and the American Jury.* Ann Arbor: University of Michigan Press.

Vietor, A. 1924. *A Woman's Quest: The Life of Marie Zakrzewska.* New York: Appleton.

Vladeck, B. 1981. "The Market vs. Regulation: The Case for Regulation." *Milbank Memorial Fund* 59(2): 209–223.

Warshaw, B. 1978. "Letter to the Editor." *Federation Bulletin* 65: 321–322.

Weiler, P. 1991. *Medical Malpractice on Trial.* Cambridge, MA: Harvard University Press.

Weir, R. 1972. "On the Antiseptic Treatment of Wounds and Its Results." *Medical America in the Nineteen Century,* ed. G. Brieger, 198–200. Baltimore: Johns Hopkins University.

West, J. 2008. "President's Message." *Federation Bulletin* 94(3): 37.

Wheeler, J. 1935. *Memoirs of a Small-Town Surgeon.* New York: Frederick Stokes.

Wielawski, I. 1986a. "Prompt Action Sought in Cases of Inept, Unethical Doctors." *Providence Journal,* January 25.

———. 1986b. "Balasco's Medical License Suspended." *Providence Journal,* January 30.

———. 1986c. "One Patient's Story." *Providence Journal,* January 30.

———. 1986d. "Medical Board Decides to Go Public with Information on Erring Doctors." *Providence Journal,* February 2.

Wieviorka, M. 2008. "Some Considerations after Reading Michael Burawoy's Article: 'What Is to Be Done? Theses on the Degradation of Social Existence in a Globalizing World.'" *Current Sociology* 56: 381–388.

Wilensky, H. 1964. "The Professionalization of Everyone?" *American Journal of Sociology* 70: 137–158.

Williams, B., and A. Matheny. 1995. *Democracy, Dialogue, and Environmental Disputes.* New Haven, CT: Yale University Press.

Williams, B., and M. Williams. 2008. "The Disruptive Physician: A Conceptual Organization." *Journal of Medical Licensure and Discipline* 94: 12–20.

Williams, G., and J. Popay. 2006. "Lay Knowledge and the Privilege of Experience." In *Challenging Medicine,* ed. D. Kelleher, J. Gabe, and G. Williams, 104–117. London: Routledge.

Wilson, J. 1978. "Interview with Dr. Wilson, Board President." *Michigan Medicine* 77 (October): 566–567.

Winn, J. 1995. "Endorsement: State vs. National Licensure." *Federation Bulletin* 82: 9–15.

Witz, A., and E. Annandale. 2006. "The Challenges of Nursing." In *Challenging Medicine*, ed. D. Kelleher, J. Gabe, and G. Williams, 23–45. London: Routledge.

Wolfe, S. 1993. "The Need for Public Access to the National Practitioner Data Bank." *Federation Bulletin* 80: 231–235.

———. 2003. "Bad Doctors Get a Free Ride." *New York Times*, March 4.

Wolfram, C. W. 1978. "Barriers to Effective Public Participation in Regulation of the Legal Profession." *Minnesota Law Review* 62: 619–647.

Wolfson, A. D., M. Trebilcock, and C. Tuohy. 1980. "Regulating the Professions: A Theoretical Framework." In *Occupational Licensure and Regulation*, ed. S. Rottenberg, 180–214. Washington, DC: American Enterprise Institute for Public Policy Research.

Wolinsky, F. 1988. "The Professional Dominance Perspective, Revisited." *Milbank Memorial Fund Quarterly* 66: 33–47.

———. 1993. "The Professional Dominance, Deprofessionalization, Proletariatization, and Corporatization Perspectives: An Overview and Synthesis." In *The Changing Medical Profession*, ed. F. W. Hafferty and J. B. McKinlay, 11–24. New York: Oxford University Press.

Wyden, R. 1993. "Health Reform, Freedom of Choice and the NPDB." *Federation Bulletin* 80(4): 224–225.

Yedidia, M. 1980. "The Lay Professional Division of Knowledge in Health Care Delivery." *Research in the Sociology of Health Care* 1: 355–377.

Yessian, M. 1994a. *CAC Workshop Proceedings* Washington, DC: CAC.

———. 1994b. "From Self-Regulation to Public Protection: Medical Licensing Authorities in an Age of Rising Consumerism." *Federation Bulletin* 81: 191–197.

Yessian, M. R., and J. M. Greenleaf. 1997. "The Ebb and Flow of Federal Initiatives to Regulate Healthcare Professionals." In *Regulation of the Healthcare Professions*, ed. T. Jost, 169–198. Chicago: Health Administration Press.

Young, I. M. 1997a. "Difference as a Resource for Democratic Participation." In *Deliberative Democracy*, ed. J. Bohman and W. Rehg, 383–406. Cambridge, MA: MIT Press.

———. 1997b. *Intersecting Voices*. Princeton, NJ: Princeton University Press.

Young, M. G. 1986. "Competence and Quality Assurance in Medicine." *Texas Medicine* 82: 64–68.

Zhou, X. 1993. "Occupational Power, State Capacities, and the Diffusion of Licensing in the American States, 1890 to 1950." *American Sociological Review* 58: 553–574.

Index

Abbott, A., 202n43, 223n5

Abel, R., 226n1

accountability: demand for, 58; lack of board, 95; of public officials, 73; public participation and, 167; and public representation, 59

administrative law judges (ALJs), 15, 225n4, 225n5; careful fact construction required by, 158; detailed opinions crafted by, 155

administrative warning, 17–18

administrators: employed by medical boards, 113; physicians as, 221n6; and role of public members, 26

Administrators in Medicine (AIM), 83

Advanced Nurse Practice Act, 118

advanced practice nurses, 92; working independently, 100–101. *See also* nurse practitioners

adverse actions, reporting, 103, 222n21. *See also* reporting

alcohol problems, among doctors, 5, 117

Alexander, E., 70

Allen, Thomas, 93

allied health professions, 61

allopathic medical societies, 37

allopaths, 34

alternative dispute resolution (ADR), 224n8

alternative medicine, 209n9. *See also* complementary medicine

altruism: in doctor-patient relationship, 226n11; professional, 56, 209n164. *See also* character issues

American Association of Medical Colleges (AAMC), 50, 201–202nn36

American Association of Retired Persons (AARP), 82–83, 214n16, 216n63

American Civil Liberties Union (ACLU), 178

American Confederation of Reciprocating, Examining, and Licensing Boards, 51

American democracy, evolving norms of, 192. *See also* democracy

American Medical Association (AMA), 34; attitude toward public members of, 63; and board accountability, 7; code of ethics of, 45, 206n107; debate about licensure, 204n81; Disabled Physician Act of, 66; doctors-to-population ratio and, 51; fear of national licensure of, 62; and FSMB, 53; and history of licensure movement, 38–39; licensure advanced by, 42, 44, 204n81; medical schools assessment of, 50; national membership of, 50; and new entry-level exam, 96; position on public members of, 7, 63; and protection of public, 45; and public participation, 61; and reform of disciplinary process, 85; on sharing of information, 84; and telemedicine practice, 95

Ameringer, C., 206n119

Andre, H. M., 90

anesthesia, 41

antiseptics: acceptance of, 42; failure to use, 41–42, 203n61

arguments: in board deliberations, 26 (*see also* deliberations, board); in IC process, 144; in sanction phase, 162–163

Arizona Republic, 81, 215n57

Astler, Vernon, 75

Atkinson, P., 206n115

autonomy, professional, 9, 169, 172

Baker, T., 227n4

Balasco, Felix, 79–80

Baltimore Sun, 93

Barger, D., 220n1

Baum, J. K., 90

Bean-Bayog, Margaret, 78

Bechamps, Gerald, 91

Benham, L., 227n36

Berlant, J., 227n35

Berman, J. I., 92

bias, and training of board members, 183

Available titles in the Critical Issues in Health and Medicine series:

About the Author

Ruth Horowitz is a professor of sociology at New York University. Her previous books include *Honor and the American Dream: Culture and Identity in a Chicano Community*, also published by Rutgers University Press (Honorable mention, C. Wright Mills Award), and *Teen Mothers: Citizens or Dependents* (Charles H. Cooley Award). Her involvement as a public member serving on a medical licensing and disciplinary board has led to her serving as a public member on the boards of several other medical organizations and a new interest in medical sociology, patient-centered medicine, and patient safety.